SLIM AFTER 40:

TAKE CONTROL
OF YOUR WEIGHT
WITHOUT DIETING

Dr Khandee Ahnaimugan

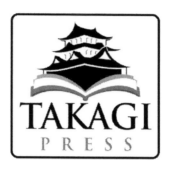

ISBN: 978-0995468207
Copyright © 2016 Dr Khandee Ahnaimugan

Published by Takagi Press
1st Printing August 2016

The information included in this book is not intended nor implied to be a substitute for professional medical advice. The reader should always consult his or her healthcare provider to determine the appropriateness of the information for their own situation or if they have any questions regarding a medical condition or treatment plan.

Also by Dr Khandee Ahnaimugan:

Slim and Healthy without Dieting:
The Definitive Weight Loss Solution for Women over 40

Losing Weight After 40:
Change Your Life Without Dieting or Deprivation

For more help on your weight loss journey, visit
www.DoctorKWeightLoss.com

.

TABLE OF CONTENTS

INTRODUCTION:
IN THE DEPTHS OF
DESPAIR, A NEW HOPE

SARAH WAS FILLED WITH DREAD as she opened her wardrobe. Although it was filled with clothes, the wardrobe might as well have been empty.

At 48 years of age, Sarah's weight had been increasing over the last few years. And today, after an invitation to dinner, she looked at her clothes and realised that only a handful of them would actually fit her.

How had it got to this?

Sarah had been on dozens of diets over the years. She had tried fasting, calorie counting, cutting out carbs and even packaged meals. She had learned about nutrition, metabolism and supplements. She had gone on boot camps and been through three personal trainers in the last five years. She had tried everything she could and yet each year her weight was going up: sometimes slowly and other times scarily fast. And now, as she stood in front of her wardrobe with a whole bunch of clothes that didn't fit, Sarah didn't know what to do next. She felt hopeless.

Sarah's story is depressingly familiar. After all, two thirds of the adult population in Western countries (and increasing percentages in the rest of the world) are either overweight or obese. In other words, more people are overweight than not.

And for women over 40, there's an added complication. Because of slowing metabolism (which happens to everyone but becomes more apparent for women after the age of 40), diets that might have worked temporarily in the past just stop working.

Even exercise becomes less and less effective.

Yes – neither diets nor exercise are enough for weight loss for women over 40.

What this means is that the two things you're "supposed" to do to lose weight don't work anymore. Is it any wonder why most women over 40 are lost about what to do next?

As options narrow, there's a sense of desperation, hopelessness and a feeling that it's only going to get worse.

When most clients first come to see me, they describe feeling totally out of control. They can't stop their weight going up and they're fresh out of ideas, because nothing has worked so far.

It's Time to Take Control

You may be fed up but you can't be completely without hope or you wouldn't be reading this! And that's great, because there *is* hope. Even if you can't rely on diets and even if exercise doesn't cut it, there is a way for women over 40 to lose weight and keep it off.

Instead of being at the mercy of a gradually increasing weight, I want to show you how you can regain control of your health by changing your relationship with food.

But the catch is that you're going to have to think differently. You won't achieve your goal with the usual diet or exercise plan. The method I'm going to tell you about in this book is a completely different way of losing weight. It's the approach that I use every day with clients at my clinic. It's how they are able to lose weight without dieting or deprivation and keep their weight off for the long-term. And now it's time for you to learn how they do it.

I often tell clients that the moment when you feel really fed up is actually the greatest point of opportunity. It's the time when you're most willing to cast aside your previously held beliefs and embrace a totally different approach.

And once you've had your mind opened in this way, it will be hard to ever go back.

How To Read This Book

In this book, I'm not only going to show you a new way of thinking about losing weight; I'm also going to equip you with the practical tools to make lasting weight loss happen in your life.

Throughout this book, I've focused on the real-life challenges of my weight-loss clients. You will see that many of these situations will be similar to challenges you may have encountered in your life. And by showing you how my clients dealt with them, I want to help you to deal with them too.

My suggestion for reading this book is: go through it once to get the overall feel. Then, after the first read, go back and re-read each chapter. Focus on the weight loss strategies mentioned in each chapter and look for how you can apply them to your life.

The way you lose weight for the long-term is by changing your habits. And this requires repetition. If you keep revisiting each chapter of this book and keep actively looking for changes you can make to your life, this will help form new habits. You will be creating a new, healthy relationship with food.

Let's face it. You're sick of dieting. You're sick of the strict eating plans. You're sick of feeling deprived and hungry and miserable. There comes a point when it's hard to keep doing the same things over and over again and still find that you're not getting anywhere.

Instead, think of a future, free of dieting. Think of a future, feeling slim and healthy for life. I'm looking forward to showing you how you can take control and make this happen in your life.

Dr Khandee Ahnaimugan MBChB MMed
London, August 2016

1

STOP BLAMING YOURSELF: THE REAL REASON YOU STRUGGLE TO LOSE WEIGHT

WHEN YOU'RE THINKING ABOUT YOUR weight, how often do you end up blaming yourself for not being able to figure it all out?

Most women I see at my clinic blame themselves for being overweight.

For example, one of my clients, Natalie, had a successful career at a publishing company as well as a close relationship with her husband and two children. But despite this, constant worrying about her weight took up a lot of her time.

Natalie told me that feeling bad about her weight was often the first thought she had in the morning; it recurred regularly throughout the day and was her last thought before she went to sleep.

She couldn't stand that this one area of her life was out of her control. And she felt like a failure because she had tried so many different ways to lose weight and still couldn't succeed. Natalie was certain there was something wrong with her and hated herself for it.

Although I understood her feelings of frustration, I would never have said that Natalie was to blame for her predicament.

This is because I knew something that she was yet to realise. The reason she had not succeeded was not because of a personal failing but simply because she had been doing the wrong things to lose weight.

She may have tried lots of different methods over the years but ultimately every single thing had been a variation on dieting.

A diet is a diet is a diet.

When it comes down to it, dieting doesn't work. I mentioned earlier why slowing metabolism makes diets less effective as you get older.

But it's more than that. Diets are fundamentally flawed.

They are drastic and unpleasant methods of losing weight. Even if you put up with the deprivation long enough to lose weight, as soon as you stop the diet and go back to old habits, your weight will come back.

Diets are a short-term solution to a long-term problem.

The upshot of this is if you haven't managed to lose weight so far, it's not because there's something wrong with you, it's because there's something wrong with dieting!

What this means is that it's time to forgive yourself. You are not flawed. You haven't done anything wrong. You are not to blame for struggling to lose weight with diets. You may have tried your best but dieting was never going to be the solution you thought it would be.

It's time to stop blaming yourself and time to focus on a more long-term sustainable method of losing weight.

Chapter Summary

1. It's not your fault if you haven't been able to manage your weight till now.

2. Most people have tried dieting to lose weight; this is ultimately doomed to failure, because it's a short-term solution to a long-term problem.

2

DON'T LOSE WEIGHT
FOR THE WRONG REASON

You only need to lose weight

for your health, wellbeing

and to get more out of life.

You don't need to lose weight

to prove anything about yourself

or what kind of person you are.

You are **OK** regardless.

3

THE OPPOSITE OF DIETING

CATH WAS GOING ON HER third diet of the year. Her aim for this one was to lose ten pounds, preferably as quickly as possible.

She knew that to achieve this, she would need to be very strict. There would be no room for chocolate or bread or pasta. And certainly no room for socialising. She would try and keep her calendar (and fridge) as empty as possible.

Unfortunately, within a few days of starting her diet, after a tough day at work and an argument with her husband, she had a blowout which ended up with her eating a large amount of chocolate.

She felt so angry with herself and fed up with the whole thing. And at the moment, her diet was over. Again.

Despite her best intentions and lots of experience with trying to lose weight, Cath was unable to succeed.

And her story is pretty common. Cath did what most people do when they try and lose weight and this was why it all went wrong.

Let's tease out Cath's example to see what she could have done differently.

1. It's not just about losing weight.

When most people think of weight loss, they understandably focus only on the *losing weight* part.

That's why you will often hear people proudly declare how much weight they lost and how quickly they did it.

For example, "I lost 10 pounds in 2 weeks".

But what's the point of losing weight, if you gain it all back a few weeks later?

Weight loss without weight maintenance is meaningless.

Your focus needs to be on how you can lose weight *and* keep it off.

As soon as you start thinking in this way, you start focusing on doing things that are sustainable, which makes all the difference.

2. Deprivation is Bad

Most people associate losing weight with deprivation and unpleasantness.

Dieting is about cutting out foods you love and missing out on enjoyable eating situations.

But as soon as losing weight becomes unpleasant, it becomes something you're only willing to do for a short time.

So, unpleasantness is not compatible with long-term weight control.

Not just that, but being forbidden from eating foods that you love increases the cravings for them. The pressure builds up and eventually the dam bursts, resulting in overeating.

Therefore, deprivation is not only unsustainable (because no one wants to suffer for the long-term), but it also makes binges more likely.

To achieve long-term weight loss, you need to be able to lose weight without feeling deprived.

Is this even possible? Yes! And you're going to learn how.

3. Dealing with Everyday Situations

Like Cath did, you're probably aware of people (you may have even done this yourself) who plan to lose weight during quiet times in their schedule. They try to lose weight between significant social events but won't ever consider it during trips away, Christmas or other holidays.

While on a weight loss programme, they may also try and avoid excessive socialising (or they get stressed out when they have to do it).

How many dinner invites have you turned down because you were trying to lose weight?

Yes, it might seem to make sense to schedule a weight loss attempt during a time when you have as few distractions as possible, but there are a few flaws to this approach.

Firstly, life is busy. It's often really difficult to find a couple of quiet weeks. Something always comes up.

Secondly, going out for dinner or going on holiday are part of a normal, enjoyable lifestyle. If you don't learn what to do (and really, how many diets even mention how to cope with these situations?), then as soon as one of these situations comes along, your efforts will be derailed.

You need to learn to master these sorts of situations, or your weight loss will always be precarious.

4. What happens when things go wrong?

The last time you went on a diet and things went wrong, you probably thought, "I've messed it all up!"

Most people associate making mistakes with failure.

But it's time to change your perspective.

With this approach, it's not about perfection. It's about persistence. As long as you persist, mistakes mean nothing. As long as each time you fall over, you stand up again, nothing can stop you.

To put it another way:

The only way you can fail with this approach is if you give up.

So just keep going!

Enjoy life and manage your weight

As far as I'm concerned, one of the most important parts of this weight loss approach is that you will be able to enjoy life and still lose weight.

I want you to be able to eat foods you like (even carbs!), go out for dinner and on holiday and still manage your weight. It's only when you can do all these things that you will stick with the plan for life.

Now, I am fully aware that the idea of being able to enjoy foods you like (from all food groups) *and* still lose weight might seem a little far-fetched.

You might even feel it's impossible. After all, it goes against everyday views of how to lose weight.

But actually, one of the best things about my job is seeing clients experience that moment of realisation that they are eating less and yet they don't feel deprived at all.

It feels like a miracle! Let me show you how it's possible…

Chapter Summary

1. Change your focus from losing weight to losing weight *and* keeping it off. This is such an important distinction.

2. Deprivation is bad! It undermines your ability to manage your weight for the long-term.

3. Rather than avoiding socialising and other enjoyable activities, it's best to learn how to handle them.

4. The only way you can fail with this approach is if you give up.

4

THE MAGIC OF THE
FOOD DIARY: PART 1

HERE ARE SOME COMMON PROBLEMS faced by dieters:

"I don't know why I'm gaining weight. I feel like I'm eating quite healthily. It must be something wrong with my metabolism."

"I know what to do but keep slipping up."

"I hate following a diet."

I have a solution for all three of these concerns: The food diary. If you've read any of my previous books, you'll know that I am a strong believer in the food diary for weight loss.

Let's look at each of these concerns in turn:

"I don't know why I'm gaining weight. I feel like I'm eating quite healthily. It must be something wrong with my metabolism."

To be blunt, impressions are worthless. You may think that your weight problems are a mystery but until you write down accurately what you are eating and drinking, you can't make any judgments about your metabolism.

Most people will find, after a week or so of keeping their food diary, that it's fairly obvious where things are going wrong.

"I know what to do but keep slipping up."

By keeping a food diary, it improves your awareness. That is a huge part of this process. Most people sleep-walk through their day when it comes to food. They have longstanding habits that they just stick to.

If you want to change, you need to introduce awareness. You need to be aware of what you're doing.

And simply by being more aware, it becomes harder to make mistakes. When you have to write down what you're eating (and ideally show it to someone else), then it can change your behaviour.

"I hate following a diet."

When you follow a diet, you are given a list of things you should and shouldn't eat. But we want to establish a more natural relationship with food. And for that we need to establish the baseline. We need to know your normal routine with food. That means keeping a food diary.

The food diary shows many things aside from what you're eating.

When you go through a food diary and ask the right questions, you figure out not just what you eat but WHY.

We'll talk more about this in the next chapter.

But keeping a food diary is a pain in the neck...

I would agree with you that keeping a food diary is annoying *if* it means weighing every item of food, counting calories, adding them up, entering into an app and so on.

But that level of detail is not necessary, unless you really feel compelled or excited by it (in that case, go for it).

At its most basic level, I would suggest taking a piece of paper and making two columns.

In the left column, write the day of the week and the date.

In the right column, write down the time and what you had to eat.

That's it.

Keep it simple. Don't give yourself an excuse to not do it.

Do I Have to Use Pen and Paper?

If you like technology and have found an app that works well for you, then that's fine. But if you find that it makes things more difficult, just stick with a notebook or a piece of paper.

I have some clients who turn up every week for their appointment with their food diary scrawled on a crumpled piece of paper. I don't mind as long as it's all there.

It's more important that the information is captured, not how it's captured.

The other thing I would suggest with food diaries is to write down what you've eaten *as soon as you can*. The longer you wait, the more likely you'll forget things. Especially snacks.

Review your food diary again at the end of the week.

It can be helpful to look over your food diary at the end of the week. We will talk more about this in the next chapter.

Chapter Summary

1. The food diary is your absolute essential tool for losing weight.

2. It keeps you aware, helps you know what is going on and helps you decide what changes to make.

3. It doesn't matter how you keep the food diary, as long as you keep it. Paper or electronic, either is OK.

4. Keep the food diary as simple as possible. If it becomes a pain in the neck, you're doing it wrong.

5

THE MAGIC OF THE
FOOD DIARY: PART 2

As we discussed in the last chapter, keeping a food diary will help you get an accurate picture of your eating and drinking.

It will also affect your behaviour if you know you have to write it down.

But with my weight loss method, the real benefit is when you analyse your food diary.

Analysing Your Own Food Diary

When you analyse your food diary, it gives you a deeper understanding of your eating patterns that you can use to make profound and lasting changes to your eating.

With clients I see at my clinic, the question I want to ask with every food decision is:

"Why did you have *that much* of *that food*, at *that time*?"

Let's break that down a bit more.

"Why did you have *that much*..."

This is all about portion sizes. Why do you choose a particular amount for breakfast, or for snacks or for dinner?

"of *that food*..."

Why do you eat cereal for breakfast? Or eggs? Most people don't even give a second thought to their routine food choices. They eat eggs for breakfast, because they've always had eggs for breakfast. (I'm not saying there's anything wrong with eggs for breakfast; I just want you to be aware of the reasons you make certain decisions.)

"at *that time*?"

What triggers you to eat at certain times? Often people eat because it's a certain time, whether they are hungry or not. Or things in their environment trigger eating, like walking past a bakery.

The question "Why did you eat that much of that food at that time?" also comes back to satisfaction. Was what you ate satisfying?

Most people don't think about this. They eat a chocolate bar, because, hey, they like chocolate. But they never think: is this flavour actually satisfying? Do I like other chocolate bars better? How do I feel afterwards?

You may think you like a particular food; however, when you *really* think about it, you realise that every time you have it, it might taste good but you feel sick afterwards.

You need to understand which foods (and drink) actually give you satisfaction and which don't.

As you ask these questions, you'll get a clearer sense of why you eat what you eat and what payoff you're getting out of it.

Changes You Can Make

Understanding food choices, food amounts and responses to the environment is absolutely essential for a non-dieting approach. When you know why you eat *that much* of *that food* at *that time*, you have some valuable information to start introducing new changes to your eating, for example:

- Perhaps that portion for lunch is too much?

- Perhaps having that orange juice for breakfast could be replaced by something better?

- Perhaps having that meal ½ hour earlier might stop snacking?

These sorts of questions are the foundation of making lasting changes, which we'll explore more throughout this book.

But you can't make these changes without the information you get from keeping a food diary.

Get someone else to look at it.

Of course, it's even more useful to get someone else to look at your food diary, because they will see things that you don't.

This means choosing the right people to help you. Most of us are victims of the "availability bias" where we pick the people who are around us (like family members or friends), because they are convenient and available. But just because they're around doesn't make them the ideal person.

Many people you ask for help, especially if they are overweight themselves, have their own baggage when it comes to weight loss. And they may also have their own theories for how to lose weight, which don't work for you.

If you're sharing your food diary, what you want to be wary of is people looking at it from a "diet" perspective. For instance, you don't want them to say, "You shouldn't have had that chocolate cake", because as you're going to see, there's nothing wrong per se with having chocolate cake.

Instead, you want them to help you spot patterns, identify triggers and keep you accountable.

For instance, if they noticed that you are having a lot of peanut butter during the day, they can point it out. There's nothing wrong with any particular decision but you want to clarify *why* you're doing it. Is it because of a deliberate decision, or is it a bad habit (or simply because it's there)?

If you can't find anyone to look at your food diary, don't worry. You can still do this yourself.

Just do it.

The biggest issue with the food diary is that it seems so simple and easy that you either don't get around to doing it or dismiss it as being too basic.

That is a big mistake.

If you had to choose only one action to do from this entire book, I would say it's keeping a food diary. It is THAT important.

Chapter Summary

1. The biggest benefit from a food diary is analysing it, based on the question *"Why did you have that much of that food at that time?"*

2. With greater understanding of your interactions with food, you can make profound changes to your diet.

6

YOU DON'T NEED TO CHANGE
EVERYTHING OVERNIGHT

IN THIS CHAPTER I'M GOING to talk about a major difference between my approach to weight loss and the standard diet. Let's look at an example.

Paula was starting a diet. She knew that she had to do something about her weight but her heart sank when she contemplated starting a diet.

Not only was it depriving but she also felt like she had to overhaul her life.

All the things she enjoyed were banned.

She didn't even have to tell her family that she was on a diet. They knew immediately, because she would stop eating the same meals as them. It happened so often nowadays, no one even commented anymore.

And her husband knew she was on a diet because of that look of terror on her face if he even mentioned a dinner invite from friends.

Dieting meant a complete suspension of normal life for Paula and she hated it.

Overnight Changes Are Too Much

One of the most unreasonable things about dieting is the requirement to completely change your eating overnight.

It doesn't matter if your usual diet is pizza, hot dogs and French fries, because starting tomorrow, you're a salad eater!

Forget what you used to enjoy eating.

Forget your usual routine.

Forget your family's routine.

And you're also expected to stick to the new plan one hundred per cent of the time. Any slip-up is considered "cheating" or even failure.

This highlights a big shortcoming of the diet approach. It's drastic and unreasonable.

After a lifetime of eating a particular way, it's difficult to change overnight.

Trying to switch what you eat without acknowledging your habits is doomed to failure.

In fact, if you look around, you'll see that more and more people are using words like "behaviour", "habits" and "lifestyle" in relation to losing weight. This was VERY uncommon even ten years ago.

There is a growing realisation that to achieve long-term results, you have to acknowledge and change habits.

How do you change habits?

In short, if you repeat a behaviour over and over again, you create a new habit.

When the new behaviour becomes automatic, it is a habit.

In these cases the new behaviour becomes effortless and sometimes even unconscious.

So our aim needs to be to create a natural transformation of habits that is easy to live with.

But if changing habits was as simple as repetition, then you'd just have to eat salad for a few weeks and eventually you'd have a habit. Obviously, this isn't how it works.

In short, the habit will only last if it easily fits into your life.

For instance, if your family eats pizza every night, you love pizza and you're the director of the local pizza appreciation society, then even if you manage to eat salad every day for two months, chances are there would be too much pressure to return to your pizza-eating ways. Most people in that situation would find it too difficult to stick to their plan.

Conventional diet-thinking would blame the person for not being motivated or lacking willpower.

But I don't see it that way. I see it that trying to change behaviour without acknowledging your old habits, likes and dislikes and the environment you live in, is doomed.

Instead we have to be pragmatic. Instead of aiming for some perfect scenario ("You will never eat pizza again"), we aim for a strategy that is most likely to work.

If your life revolves around pizza, we have to figure out how you can occasionally eat pizza and still achieve your weight goals.

So this speaks to a hugely important part of this process. The changes we make have to be sustainable.

Chapter Summary

1. If you want long-term results, you need to change your habits.

2. Habits happen through repetition of behaviours but especially when we ensure that the new habits fit into your existing lifestyle.

7

THE GOLDEN QUESTION

IN THIS CHAPTER I'M GOING to teach you something that will totally change your interaction with food.

It's something that every client who sees me at my clinic learns about. In fact it's one of the first things I teach them.

It's called the Golden Question.

When you learn the Golden Question and apply it to your life, it will give you back control over your behaviour. It will give you a compass for guiding your decisions about what to eat and what not to eat. You will be able to handle any situation and know what to do. Food and cravings will no longer have a control over you and you will no longer feel guilt and self-blame associated with eating.

If you've ever had that battle in your head about whether you should eat something or not, asking the

Golden Question will give you the answer you need. It will help you to eat less without feeling deprived.

When I get feedback from clients about which parts of my approach made the biggest difference to their lives, they often tell me it's the Golden Question.

Equally, when clients feel that they are drifting off track, it's because they have been forgetting to ask the Golden Question.

So here's the question that will change how you make food decisions:

"I can have it if I want to, but do I really need it right now?"

The Two Parts of the Golden Question

The question has two equally important parts. The first part is letting you know an important aspect of this eating philosophy.

"I can have it if I want to..."

You can have *whatever you want*. Yes, that's right; you're allowed to eat whatever you want. Nothing is forbidden. I don't want you to feel that any food is off-limits. As we talked about earlier, making foods forbidden just increases the cravings for them.

What you choose to eat is in your control.

"But do I really need it right now?"

The second part of the question – "but do I really need it right now?" – is the proviso. You can have whatever you want but you have to determine whether you really need it right now.

What do I mean by *need?*

When I say need, I don't mean just reducing food down to how much you need to survive. I also mean need in terms of enjoyment. Food tastes good! Don't ignore that!

You want to be able to eat food to be nourished. But you also want to eat food to feel satisfied.

When something is neither nutritious nor enjoyable, then it is not needed. I call this the *magic margin*. If you eliminate the magic margin (food that is neither enjoyable nor nutritious), you can eat less without feeling deprived.

The Golden Question in Action

Let's look at a practical example:

You've just had dinner and some dessert at a restaurant. The waiter brings you the bill with some small, wrapped chocolates on the tray.

"I can have it if I want to, but do I really need it right now?"

Instead of saying to yourself "I'm not allowed to have chocolate", which immediately makes the chocolate more alluring, you say to yourself, "I can have it if I want to", because guess what? You can. You have the freedom to eat whatever you want.

"But do I really need it right now?"

You just had dessert! Do you really need this chocolate right now? If you think about it, you realise that you don't. You're allowed to eat it but you don't need it. So you say, "thanks but no thanks" and leave the chocolates on the tray.

The Golden Question enables you to prioritise every food decision, to improve your awareness of your food decisions and to make better decisions, without feeling deprived.

What If I Ask the Golden Question And End Up Saying Yes?

Always remember, with a question like this ("I can have it if I want to, but do I really need it right now?"), sometimes the answer can be: "Yes, I do need it right now!" and that's OK. In those cases, you should be able to eat it without guilt.

As with anything, the more you ask the question, the more it will become second nature and easier to do.

You will see, as you ask the Golden Question, that much of your eating is actually unnecessary. By asking the question, you are identifying and eliminating unnecessary eating and thereby eating less without feeling deprived.

Chapter Summary

1. The Golden Question "I can have it if I want to, but do I really need it right now?" is the key to handling any eating situation.

2. If a food is neither nutritious nor enjoyable, it is unnecessary. This unnecessary food is the "magic margin" in your eating and if you eliminate the magic margin, you can eat less and therefore lose weight without feeling deprived.

8

WHY BEING ALLOWED
TO EAT WHAT YOU WANT
WON'T LEAD TO DISASTER

IN THE LAST CHAPTER I told you that you can eat whatever you want and still lose weight.

How does that feel?

When I told one of my clients, Sally, about the Golden Question, she said that this kind of eating freedom terrified her.

That's a very common response.

After years of diet brainwashing, it's easy to see why you might not "trust" yourself to be given the freedom to eat what you want. In fact it might sound like a disaster waiting to happen.

You might imagine that if you're allowed to eat whatever you want, you'd end up eating hundreds of cakes, bars of chocolate and packets of biscuits. It's why many women I see in my clinic tell me that they have only ever felt "safe" on a regime of some sort.

But as I could see from Sally's example, her eating life had become either:

a) "I'm on a regime".

or

b) "I'm rebelling against the regime".

or

c) "I'm feeling depressed that I can't stick to a regime".

The regime feels like the safe option but it's actually the most dangerous.

If I tell you not to scratch your nose, what do you feel like doing? You get a sudden overwhelming urge to scratch your nose! And if I tell you that you can't eat chocolate ever again, it makes you desire it even more. You want to rebel.

And no matter how good you are, eventually there will be an opportunity to eat the forbidden foods.

For women who are on a strict regime, when they rebel, it often snowballs because they have thoughts like:

"I'll just eat it today and start being good again tomorrow" or "I'd better indulge as much as possible because it's back to suffering when I restart the regime".

Even if you don't consciously have those thoughts, they are probably in the back of your mind somewhere.

This sort of overeating is reactionary. It's not based on your actual hunger or desire. It's going giddy with freedom, because you've been constrained on a stifling regime.

Free Yourself

Most of the women I meet who feel like they need to be on a regime are usually *gaining* weight overall. In other words, even though they feel like a regime is necessary, it's not working for them.

So why do they stick with it? Because they fear that without the regime, their weight would increase even more.

But actually, the opposite is true.

Once you free yourself of the regime, you actually reduce the reactionary eating.

If you know that you can eat things you like whenever you want and you're not going back to a strict regime, it reduces the need to binge.

So for most women, the diet regime that seems like it's helping them is actually hurting them.

And let's face it: women who are naturally slim don't rely on regimes. It's all about natural eating.

It Takes a Leap of Faith

The problem is that abandoning an eating regime can be quite difficult to do. Most women find it terrifying because sticking to a strict eating plan is what they've always been told to do to lose weight.

To give it up requires a leap of faith.

As difficult as it may seem, part of the journey of losing weight and keeping it off means releasing yourself from the shackles of a regime and giving yourself the freedom to eat what you want.

This can be scary but once you get used to it, it is liberating.

Chapter Summary

1. Although it can feel dangerous to give yourself freedom to eat what you want, it's the restriction of eating that drives your cravings.

2. When you stop making food forbidden, it reduces much of the hold it had on you.

9

WHICH IS BETTER?
THE CHOCOLATE
OR THE APPLE?

A CLIENT (LET'S CALL HER SOPHIE) went to a country fair one weekend. Sophie had just signed up for my weight loss programme but had not yet started her sessions.

Sophie went to this fair every year and every year she looked forward to eating a particular chocolate dessert that was only available there. This year, however, Sophie had second thoughts. After all, she had just signed up for a weight loss programme and it seemed ridiculous to be indulging.

However, in the end she couldn't resist and ended up ordering one of the desserts and sharing it with her husband. She ate each mouthful with gusto. It was delicious.

And yet afterwards Sophie felt extremely guilty, because it was quite chocolatey and certainly could not be classified as "healthy".

What Would You Have Done?

How do you feel about this example? Would you have had the chocolate dessert at all, knowing that you were meant to be starting a weight loss programme in a few days?

Would you have gritted your teeth and resisted it? If you had resisted it, would you have felt virtuous that you were doing the right thing? Perhaps you may have tried to resist it but then given in, cursing yourself much like my client had?

Or would you have eaten it as part of your last hurrah, squeezing in some final bits of indulgence before the weight loss begins, knowing that it was wrong but doing it anyway?

Before I talk more about this, let's look at another example.

Denise and the Apple

Another client, let's call her Denise, was at home. She had eaten a very heavy lunch and had been doing some work at the kitchen table.

After about an hour, she decided to take a break. Denise was tempted for a second to get a cookie from the pantry but instead she had an apple while she thumbed through a magazine.

She was still quite full from the lunch and the apple was not that good but she finished it.

She was happy that she picked the apple over the cookie, congratulating herself for the decision. After all, she was trying to lose weight, so she should be eating healthily.

Who has been "good"?

From the traditional diet perspective, Sophie was "bad" for eating chocolate whereas Denise was "good" for eating fruit.

In fact, I bet you've had situations in the past, when you felt guilty for eating chocolate and virtuous for choosing fruit over chocolate. And from a dieting point of view, that's right. But with my weight loss approach, it's wrong.

So let's look at each situation and decide who really made the best decision.

Sophie ate chocolate. But so what? Indulgence isn't a crime. I want you to be able to enjoy yourself every now and then.

I want you to break the association in your mind that losing weight requires absolute deprivation.

So in Sophie's example, she was looking forward to the dessert. She shared it with her husband and she loved it. She enjoyed every bite that she had. What's wrong with that? Nothing.

Just because it was chocolate doesn't make it a bad decision.

If she had said "I didn't enjoy it that much" or "The last few mouthfuls were awful" or "I wasn't even hungry", then that's a different story.

Now, contrast Sophie's chocolate dessert with Denise's apple.

Denise was actually full when she ate the apple.

Denise also subconsciously thought of the fruit as being a non-calorie snack because she perceived it as healthy. But even if something is healthy, you should avoid eating it mindlessly. And just because something is healthy doesn't mean it's calorie-free. This is especially true of fruit since they are high in sugar, hence calories.

Denise really didn't need to eat the apple but she did. And she didn't enjoy it. These are all things I don't want you to do.

In this example, it was actually less about the actual foods being eaten and more about the circumstances in which they were eaten.

Sophie ate what she ate because she felt like it and she only ate as much as needed to enjoy it. This would have been a good decision whether it was chocolate or an apple.

Denise ate even though she was full, even though it didn't taste good and to occupy time. Whether she ate an apple, a stick of celery or a huge chocolate dessert, it was a bad decision.

When you make eating decisions for the right reasons, you are on the right track. And as always, your filter for whether it's the right decision is the Golden Question: "I can have it if I want to, but do I really need it right now?"

Chapter Summary

1. It's OK to eat chocolate. It's not a crime! It doesn't mean you're not serious about losing weight.

2. Fruit is good for you but it's still high in calories and shouldn't be eaten mindlessly.

3. Sensible eating in many cases comes down to whether you ate something for the right reasons. You know it's a good reason if you used the Golden Question to decide if you were on the right track.

10

EVERYTHING YOU NEED TO KNOW ABOUT WEIGHING YOURSELF

(This chapter is based on an article I wrote for my website.)

Let's take a small detour now and talk about the practical side of losing weight without dieting.

Something we do need to talk about is weighing yourself.

Do you have a love-hate relationship with the scales?

When I see clients at my weight loss clinic for the first time, many also have a very complicated relationship with the weighing scales. Some weigh themselves regularly, hating the results. Others are living in a cocoon of denial, not having weighed themselves for months.

And in fact, when they arrive at my clinic, part of their anxiety has to do with stepping on the scales.

They are taken aback when I tell them that I won't be weighing them today – or ever.

What?!

Why not?

I Didn't Used to Advocate Weighing

My relationship with the scales is also somewhat complicated.

I used to think that when it came to weight loss, that scales were bad.

I used to think that frequent weighing was a sign of an unhealthy relationship with weight. After all, surely the best signs of progress are natural things like your clothes fitting better?

But I've since completely changed my mind about this.

The reasons I believe that regular weighing is helpful:

1. It's motivating.

It's actually good to get regular positive feedback about your weight. It helps to maintain motivation on the weight loss journey.

Yes, clothes fitting better is a good sign but weighing provides a more objective measure.

And while clothes fitting differently might take weeks before it shows, we need more immediate feedback to gauge whether we are on the right track.

2. It's important for weight maintenance.

Once you've reached your weight loss goal, regular weighing is very important for weight maintenance (I'll explain why later).

So if I think weighing is a good thing, then why don't I weigh clients at my clinic?

Why I don't weigh clients at my clinic

The problem with weighing at the clinic is that there are too many variables that change from week to week.

For instance, each time my clients see me, they are wearing different clothes (which will weigh different amounts). At one appointment, they may have just eaten, whereas at another they may have not had anything for several hours. They might be bursting to go to the toilet on one day (and therefore have a full bladder, which weighs more than an empty one) and not on another.

All of these factors (plus many more) affect weight and therefore make weighing at the clinic too inconsistent. You need to be consistent when you weigh yourself.

Before and After Weighing

When I used to weigh clients at the clinic, they would arrive, anxious about what the scales would show and whether the reading would back up what the scales said at home (or betray them altogether). They were concerned about whether the weight would reflect the effort they had put in all week or make it all seem worthless? The time before weighing became dominated by this anxiety and so the client would be too preoccupied to engage properly with the session.

After weighing, if the scales showed a "good" result, the client would be happy and the session could proceed as planned. But if it showed a "bad" result, they would be deflated and disappointed, which affected the rest of the session.

I mention this because it is similar to someone at home weighing herself once a week.

When you weigh yourself once a week, all of the week's efforts get focused on one weight reading. The one weight measurement takes on an unnatural significance that becomes stressful.

Just like my clinic clients judging the whole week based on what their weight was at a single moment in my clinic, I think weekly weighing, even at home, is too infrequent.

Does Weight Fluctuate Day-to-Day?
Yes.

Even with all your best efforts to standardise the weighing procedure, weight fluctuates for all sorts of reasons other than what you ate. This includes, amongst other things:

- Hydration levels

- Hormonal fluctuations

- Fluid retention

- Salt intake

- Bowel contents

- Bladder contents

This is something that everyone acknowledges but they still don't make allowance for it. When they step on the scales and the number is up, they blame their eating and themselves.

The practical implication of this is that, because of these fluctuations, one weight reading means nothing. And this is why a weekly weight reading can be totally unrepresentative.

So How Often Should I Weigh Myself?

Weight fluctuations during a typical week can be up to 4-5 pounds. If you are only weighing yourself once a week, you could easily catch the wrong extreme and get a skewed perception of progress. This becomes even more important when you're maintaining weight.

However weighing more than once a day becomes obsessive and as I mentioned, gets affected by meals. You always weigh more at the end of the day than at the beginning.

So I believe that weighing yourself once a day is ideal.

Also, when you've reached your ideal weight, daily weighing becomes your early-warning system. It's a day-to-day feedback mechanism. The biggest danger when you're at your ideal weight is little things creeping in, which you don't notice. You don't want to wait till your jeans don't fit anymore to figure out that you've gained weight. That's leaving it too late.

With daily weighing, you can respond within a few days and do something about it.

Which Scales Should I Use?

I don't mind which scales you use as long as you use the same ones each time. As you may know, different scales will deliver different results. You might find that your scales at home give you a different weight to the one at the gym. The important thing isn't the actual weight it shows but how it changes over time as you lose weight. We care more about the trend.

What's The Best Way to Weigh Myself?

Do these four things:

1. Try and weigh yourself first thing in the morning before you've had anything to eat or drink.

2. Empty your bladder and bowels.

3. Don't wear any clothes or heavy jewellery.

4. Make sure the scales are on a level surface.

Try and keep this consistent every time you weigh yourself. Record the result in your food diary. When you record the results, you will be able to notice patterns and reassure yourself that weight fluctuations are normal. The more comfortable you can get with weight fluctuations the better.

Is My Weight Affected the Next Day by What I Ate the Day Before?

I've seen enough food diaries to know that what you eat the day before has minimal relation to the weight reading the next day. For every food diary where someone eats a lot and the weight goes up the next day, I've also seen the opposite (where the weight goes down even after overeating the previous day).

Generally, I've noticed that it takes a couple of days for weight to react to what you've been eating.

What Are The Drawbacks of Daily Weighing?

The biggest drawback of daily weighing (in the early stages of losing weight) is that you take weight readings too personally and attach too much importance to them.

As I have said, each reading on its own means nothing. Because there are so many reasons for weight to fluctuate, one reading cannot give you enough information to get happy or sad.

If you don't take this on board, you may end up riding the daily weight emotional roller coaster.

When the weight is down, you feel like you're doing well and life is good.

When the weight is up or stays the same, you feel despondent, like your weight loss is going nowhere and that life is terrible.

Because weight is so variable day-to-day, you can't allow each reading to affect you in this way. At my clinic, part of my job early on is to help clients to get used to these fluctuations. When a client says to me, "My weight was up on Saturday and I was OK with it", then I know that we have made some serious progress.

The scales are not your enemy. They provide a valuable measure of progress and can be your early-warning system once you've lost weight. Developing a healthy relationship with the scales can be an important part of your success.

Chapter Summary:

1. Get comfortable with the benefits of weighing yourself every day. It's a good way of measuring progress.

2. Once you're maintaining your weight, daily weighing is your early-warning system.

3. Weigh yourself at roughly the same time of day, each day and write down the results.

4. Weigh yourself free of all "excess baggage", i.e. naked with empty bladder and bowels.

5. Never take one reading too seriously. Accept that weight fluctuates for everyone, every day. Don't ride the daily-weight emotional roller coaster.

11

HOW PEOPLE WHO
EAT HEALTHILY CAN STILL
BECOME OVERWEIGHT

HERE IS A QUESTION I'm often asked: "I eat healthily and I still can't lose weight. Is there something wrong with me?"

This is a very common situation. First of all, it should be noted that if you are having trouble losing weight, it's important to get things checked out with your family doctor, especially looking for any medical conditions that might affect your weight. This is not common but worth excluding. Also some medicines, can cause weight gain or make weight loss more difficult.

On the other hand, for the vast majority of women, there won't be a medical cause and so it might seem like a mystery as to why healthy eating doesn't lead to weight loss.

It's easy to think that if someone is overweight, that they are mainly eating foods like pizza, hamburgers and French fries. These are high calorie foods and it's not surprising if you eat these regularly that you might struggle to manage your weight.

But it's a misconception that the only way to get overweight is by eating lots of fast foods and high calorie snacks. There are plenty of people who eat "healthily" and yet they are still overweight.

There are three things we need to look at.

What Does Eating Healthily Even Mean?

Firstly, we need to figure out what "eating healthily" means.

There are so many different food philosophies today, preaching different versions of health, that you would be forgiven for feeling confused.

Is eating carbs unhealthy? Is eating fat unhealthy?

Put a different way, I think most of us can recognise a blatantly unhealthy diet: large quantities of processed foods. But it's harder to see what is specifically healthy.

And you can also consume large amounts of calories from foods that you might have thought were healthy (fruit is the prime example).

The Problem With Eating Healthily Most of the Time

Secondly, often clients will tell me that they eat healthily "most of the time".

Even if you eat healthily most of the time, you can do lots of damage in *the rest of the time.*

Most people are not really aware of how many calories they're actually consuming (for example, alcohol – which people are encouraged to drink for heart health – is basically liquid calories).

Again, this is why a food diary is so important, because it helps you figure out what's actually happening, as opposed to a vague impression that you're eating healthily.

The Non-Obvious Way You're Gaining Weight

And lastly, a lot of the damage is done in small increments.

Over time, small increases in portion size can have significant effects on weight.

What this comes down to is that the habits that cause you to gain weight are not as obvious as you might think.

Let's take the example of breakfast. Let's say you've always had a bowl of cereal for breakfast since your twenties. If you're 50 now, you may have inadvertently increased the portions of cereal by 20% in that time. This can so easily happen. And even such a small increase in calories can result in a few extra pounds over a year or so.

Not just that, but did you know that a woman in her fifties may require 400 fewer calories per day than a woman in her twenties? That means if you eat as much when you are 55 as you did when you were 25, you'll be getting 400 more calories than you need. And so you'll be gaining weight.

Even if you kept eating the same things, as you get older, you will be in calorie excess and therefore gain weight.

This is just from something as innocuous as breakfast.

Multiply this throughout the day and you can see how, despite thinking that you're being healthy and not eating "bad" food, you can still be gaining weight.

Now you could hear this, as many women do and think, "That's so depressing! Even if I eat just 20% more cereal, over time it's going to add pounds to my weight!" But it also works the other way too. You don't need to make massive changes to your eating to lose weight. Cutting back a little bit, over lots of different parts of your diet, will add up over time.

Chapter Summary

1. Although it seems like it should be the answer, eating healthily doesn't necessarily mean you will be losing weight.

12

A QUICK WAY TO TELL
IF A WEIGHT LOSS PLAN
WON'T WORK

WHAT DOES IT TAKE TO manage your weight for the long-term?

The people who succeed at losing weight are the ones who develop a

- Sustainable

- System

The "system" part refers to a set of strategies.

If you open a magazine, surf the net or talk to your friends, you will find lots of systems. For example: don't eat gluten, don't eat carbs, don't eat sugar, count points, go on fasts.

But a system on its own is not enough.

For a system to be successful at weight management it must be sustainable.

The sustainable part is about doing things in a way that you can live with forever.

Will the system work for the rest of your life, and will you be able to live with it?

For instance, if your "system" for dealing with emotional eating is "just don't do it", then you are in trouble. This is not a workable or sustainable solution and you will continue to be dragged down by episodic emotion-driven eating.

Similarly, if your system for dealing with going out for dinner or on holiday is just "don't go", then how long-lasting will this be?

And if you need to resort to fasting to manage your weight but you hate fasting, then don't kid yourself. It's not a long-term plan.

I am a strong believer that every thing you do to lose weight must be something you're willing and able to do for the rest of your life. This seems obvious but how many diets have you been on where this simple idea was missing?

You must always be thinking of sustainability. And always be thinking of the long-term.

With every change you make to your eating and drinking, think: "Can I do this forever?" If not, find a different change to make.

Chapter Summary

1. Success at losing weight requires a system that is sustainable.

2. Sustainability means that whatever changes you make, you're willing to do them for the rest of your life.

13

HOW TO RESIST TEMPTATION

Temptation can feel like one of the biggest obstacles to weight loss.

Let's look at the example of one my clients (let's call her Alison).

Alison got home and saw a box of chocolates on the kitchen bench top. She remembered that she had bought the chocolates for a friend she was meeting up with for coffee. But the friend had cancelled and so Alison had brought the chocolates home.

Alison had been losing weight using my method for a few weeks, so she felt like she was on a roll. And she thought that resisting the chocolate would be a great test of her resolve.

She lasted about twenty minutes before deciding she could have one. She justified it by saying that I had told her she could "eat whatever she wanted".

One chocolate led to two, to three and eventually the whole packet was gone.

Lack of Willpower Wasn't the Problem

If Alison had been on a diet, she would have berated herself for not being able to resist the chocolate. She would have concluded that she was severely lacking in willpower and that she was never going to succeed.

You may have experienced something like this on a diet and told yourself the same things.

If *you're on a diet* and you stray off the path, you are bad! With a diet, you're expected to stick to it 100% and if you don't, you're a failure.

But I take a different view.

Every week, I have clients come in to see me after scenarios like this and instead of saying, "You were bad, try harder next time", I tease out the situation and work out what went wrong and how to avoid it happening again.

Let's break this situation down and figure out where Alison went wrong. Just to foreshadow, I don't think it was because of lack of willpower.

1. Buying chocolates that you like.

Alison did buy these chocolates for a friend not herself. But the fact is, there is always a chance the friend might cancel (as she did). Instead of buying chocolate that you like, why not buy a type of chocolate that you're not that keen on?

That way, even if you don't end up giving them to your friend, the chocolates aren't so tempting.

2. Not getting rid of the chocolates as soon as the coffee was cancelled.

Bringing the chocolates home and not getting rid of them quickly was really the biggest mistake of all.

As soon as her friend cancelled, Alison shouldn't have brought the chocolates into her house. They immediately created unnecessary temptation. Remember, if they weren't in the house it's very unlikely that Alison would have left home to buy those chocolates to eat.

In other words, she only ate them because she brought them into the house, making them completely unnecessary calories.

3. Seeing the chocolates and then not moving them out of sight.

In the fantastic book *Mindless Eating: Why We Eat More Than We Think*, Brian Wansink describes how he and his team at the Cornell Food and Brand Laboratory ran a whole host of experiments that showed that if food is in front of you and in your line of sight, you are more likely to eat it.

Each time you look at the food, you have a conversation about whether to eat it or not. And even if you only cave in once out of every ten times you will end up eating more than if the food wasn't there.

4. Describing chocolates as "bad."

Remember, as soon as you forbid yourself from having a particular food, you are intensifying your desire for it.

Food is neither good nor bad. It is just food.

If a food is "banned", you end up eating more of it, because you think, "This is my last chance".

Forget Willpower – It's All About Controlling Your Environment

So the cure for this sort of incident isn't more willpower but better control of your environment. When you take control of your environment, you are no longer at the mercy of food. And even with foods you love, you should make eating them a deliberate choice. It should be a proper decision, not just "because it was there".

When you see that your environment rather than willpower is key, you don't need to feel so discouraged when things go wrong like in this situation with Alison.

The things that will prevent this situation happening again (or at least minimising the chances of it happening again) are pretty simple. And over time, they will be easy for you to implement.

So this re-frames the entire incident. Instead of being a sober reminder of your failings, it becomes a good learning experience to highlight areas that could be improved.

Incidentally, even clients who have used my weight loss approach for years can fall into the trap of inadvertently letting foods into their home that can undermine their efforts. This is something you need to be vigilant about on an ongoing basis.

Chapter Summary

1. When you buy tempting foods, buy flavours that other people like but you don't.

2. Guard your home environment. Don't needlessly bring in tempting foods.

3. If tempting food is in your house, keep it out of sight.

4. Calling certain foods bad just intensifies the cravings for them.

5. More willpower isn't the solution to temptation. Instead, get better at controlling your environment.

14

HOW TO CUT BACK WHAT YOU'RE EATING WITHOUT FEELING DEPRIVED

SOME PEOPLE THINK THAT THEY can manage their weight, simply by having a list of foods they're not allowed to eat.

But I believe that restricting foods is a path to failure because it is depriving and can create cravings.

Instead of focusing on banning types of food, I prefer to focus on portions.

The thing I find as I go through the process of weight loss with a client is that most of us have ended up with portions that are larger than what we need – not just from a health and nutrition point of view but even from an enjoyment point of view. Portion sizes can easily creep up over the years and have no connection to actual enjoyment.

When you eat more, you *get used to* eating more.

But if you start cutting back portions, you will actually notice that you need less and less.

I notice with some clients that, seven or eight weeks into the process, they are actually eating half of what they were eating before.

Imagine that. You could be *needlessly* eating double the amount you actually need to feel satisfied.

How to Reduce Portion Sizes

The main rule in reducing portions sizes is to go slow.

I recently had a client who decided to cut portions by 50%. That's too much! She felt hungry and deprived and it was counter-productive.

I recommend starting with as little as 5%. If you usually have 20 small potatoes for dinner, it means removing one. Yes, it's a tiny amount. But that's the point. It shouldn't be noticeable. Over time, you can slowly keep reducing even more.

But always be on the lookout for how you feel. If you're still really hungry straight after the meal, you've cut back too much. Gradual change is the key. And I find for most clients, it's really freeing to be given "permission" by me to cut back that slowly. It takes the pressure off and ensures that they don't feel deprived.

And this leads back to what we described in the chapter on the Golden Question. You *don't* need to suffer to lose weight. In fact, if you are suffering, you are doing it wrong; suffering undermines your ability to stick with the plan for the long-term.

And that rule is highly relevant to how fast you cut back portions.

Be gentle and do it slowly.

Chapter Summary

1. Rather than banning whole food groups, you are better off cutting back portions.

2. Don't cut back too quickly. Start slow and go slow. If you feel hungry or deprived, you've cut back too much too soon.

15

BE GENTLE ON YOURSELF
BUT DON'T BE A VICTIM

ONE OF THE IMPORTANT PARTS of this weight loss approach is being gentle and forgiving with yourself. If you're used to being pilloried and abused by personal trainers or nutritionists for not doing enough or not wanting this enough, then this gentler approach might feel great (or a bit unusual!).

The truth is, if you do things in a sustainable way, you won't need a sergeant-major type standing over you, making you feel bad for having French fries or chocolate.

But just because we are being gentle on ourselves, does not mean we can give up all responsibility. You are still responsible for your body and what you put into it.

For example, do any of these comments sound familiar to you?

"They were having a birthday party at work, so I couldn't avoid having cake".

"I had a viral infection so I just needed the energy (that's why I ate the chocolate)".

"The dessert was just irresistible".

Now I'm not saying that external factors do not affect eating. They do. Stress, tiredness and temptation can all make us eat more than we need (or want). But the wrong response is to shrug your shoulders as if you're powerless, use it as an excuse and make no attempt to change it.

Acting like a victim will not help.

If you want to be slim and healthy for life, then you're going to have to think about how you can modify your response to these external triggers.

You have to be proactive.

Let's look at each of the scenarios:

"They were having a birthday party at work, so I couldn't avoid having cake".

It's OK to eat cake if you wanted it and enjoyed every mouthful. But this statement shows more of a case of obligation eating. Eating to please others is not a reason to eat.

"I had a viral infection so I just needed the energy (that's why I ate the chocolate)".

Re-consider your food choices for energising yourself. Why does it have to be food? And why does it have to be chocolate?

When a client complains of tiredness, we look for ways to energise themselves without resorting to food.

And I always tell them to get more sleep!

"The dessert was just irresistible".

This comment suggests a feeling of powerlessness in the face of something that tastes good.

If something really is irresistible to you, then reduce your exposure to it. In a previous chapter, we talked about how the environment affects what and how much you eat (if something is not there, you can't eat it).

I want you to be able to enjoy life and eat and drink the things you want. But this process also requires you to be proactive.

You must always be looking for ways to improve your responses to eating and drinking triggers. There is no room for passivity or excuses. You must take control.

Chapter Summary

1. There are lots of things that might happen that lead you to eating more. But you don't need to be a victim. Look for ways to proactively deal with them. This approach to weight loss is about you taking control.

16

HOW TO EAT AT
RESTAURANTS WITHOUT
GOING OVERBOARD

MANY OF THE CLIENTS WHO attend my clinic dine out regularly.

And when they do eat out, they are often thinking: "This meal costs a lot, so I want to get my money's worth".

Incidentally, this is true, whether the client is fabulously wealthy, whether their company is paying for the meal or even if it's an included breakfast at a hotel.

And often they don't even realise that they're having that thought or that it's affecting how much they eat.

It doesn't matter how much the meal costs; most of us have these thoughts in our head because most of us associate value with having more (everyone loves Happy Hour!). And when you're eating at a restaurant, it's natural to think that having more is how you get the full value out of the experience.

But let's take a step back.

The Question to Ask

What is the real value of eating at a restaurant?

For many people, on an unconscious level, getting value means:

- Eating nice food.
- Eating as much as possible.
- Eating as many different things as possible.

By this reasoning, instead of going out for dinner, if I locked you in a padded room on your own and had a conveyor belt deliver you masses of quality food, you would be equally happy.

But of course, there's much more to eating out than that. When you go to a restaurant to eat, you're enjoying:

- The ambience.
- The decor.
- A night out.
- Socialising.
- Not having to cook the meal.
- Being served by someone else.
- The presentation of the food.

That list of reasons, you'll note, has little to do with eating vast amounts of food.

What we really need to focus on is satisfaction. That is the real measure of value. Not how much you eat.

Can you feel satisfied with fewer courses? Probably.

By societal convention, most of us tend to order a starter, a main course and a dessert. But realistically, most of us only need two courses to feel happy.

Is it more satisfying to finish a meal not feeling bloated, sick or uncomfortably full? Yes, of course.

If you get to the end of the meal feeling satisfied and having had a good time, then that is a good meal.

What this means is reconsidering what you think of as enjoyment. You're trying to have a pleasant, memorable night out. Eating so much you need to have your stomach pumped shouldn't be part of the deal.

When you think about dinners at restaurants as more about the other aspects of going out than about the food, you can't help but eat less (and enjoy it more, because you're not overfull).

Chapter Summary

1. The point of eating out is not to eat as much as possible.

2. Shift the emphasis onto feeling satisfied during and *after* the meal.

3. This means focusing on non-food aspects of eating out, like the night out, the restaurant environment and the people you're with.

17

A TEST FOR YOU

HERE'S A TEST FOR YOU, to see if you're really committed to this new way of thinking about managing your weight.

Imagine you're at a party. You're talking to a friend and the topic turns to weight.

Your friend tells you: "I just lost five pounds in one week on this amazing new diet".

What's your response?

Do you want to find out more about this diet, because you might want to go on it? After all, you wouldn't mind losing five pounds in a week, right?

While it might seem impressive at first glance, your friend losing five pounds in a week is not much of an achievement if she gains it all back a few weeks later. What is important is that your friend is able to stick with it.

And how do you work out if a particular weight loss method is sustainable?

Here are some things to look out for (Compare it to any diets you've been on in the past).

- Does it require lots of preparation and planning? If so, it's less sustainable.

- Does following it mean that you have to be very strict and not eat things you like? This is not sustainable.

- Is it unpleasant? This is definitely not sustainable. Who wants to be miserable for the rest of their life?

- Do you feel like you could only really stay on the regime for a few weeks? This probably sums up most diets and it's, of course, not sustainable.

There Will Always Be a Temptation to Go For a Quick Fix

When you're using my approach to weight loss and focused on lifestyle change, you will be tempted by diets and weight loss plans promising quick results.

I have one client who would turn up every week, telling me about how a different friend had lost weight on some short-term disaster diet and how tempted she was to try it.

She ended up losing one and a half stone (22 pounds) using my method and without having to resort to dieting. But I have to say, for her, the temptation to chase a diet was there almost till the end.

Even though she was steadily losing weight without feeling deprived, she still felt tempted because these diets promise a fantasy quick fix. Even if it's not sustainable and even if they have never, ever worked for you.

There's no shortage of people you know who will have fallen under the spell of a crash diet and you'll probably catch them just as they're going through a temporary high because they've lost a few pounds quickly. But it doesn't last. You know that! That's why you're reading this book.

You need to see past the superficial. You need to resist the temptation to go back to the dark side. Leave the short-term diets to people who don't know any better and stick with your focus on long-term weight control.

Chapter Summary

1. Although it might seem tempting, there is nothing to be gained from trying a diet.

2. Fight the temptation to chase after the newest diet and focus on long-term lifestyle change instead. You know it's the right decision.

18

THE WRONG KIND
OF OPTIMISM: PART 1

O FTEN WHEN TRYING TO LOSE weight, it can be easy to gloss over potential problems that will come up. There can be a lot of reasons for doing this but the main one is to avoid thinking.

> *"Thinking is the hardest work there is, which*
> *is probably the reason why so few engage in it."*
>
> – Henry Ford

It's easier to just push on, instead of stepping back and thinking about the course of action you're embarking on. After all, if most people going on a diet spent even ten minutes thinking about what they were doing, they would see that it wasn't sustainable and unlikely to deliver the result they desired.

A good example is people who go on diets where the meals are delivered to their house. It's pretty clear that unless you're willing to eat packaged meals for the rest of your life, it's not a long-term solution. (And what do you do when you go on holiday?)

A common rationalisation is "I'll just lose the weight first and then worry about how I'm going to keep it off". But this doesn't work, because even if you manage to lose weight, you will struggle to maintain your weight loss.

If you have embraced my weight loss approach, it is still possible to make mistakes by hoping for the best instead of doing the work of figuring out how to cope with a challenging situation.

In my book *Losing Weight after 40*, I mentioned the example of a client heading for a holiday to Australia and saying, "It's warm there, so I should be OK". This is crazy, because there are as many overweight and obese people in Australia as there are in the UK. Warm climates don't prevent weight gain.

Another common example of foolish optimism is when clients are going to a buffet dinner. They know there will be a lot of food and a lot of temptation and their plan is "I will just have to be restrained".

First of all, restraining yourself is too diet-y. I want you to enjoy life, not feel restrained. Restrained = deprivation = more cravings = impending doom.

Secondly, "I just have to be restrained" is not a sustainable strategy. You might be able to do this now, while you're fired up and eager to lose weight. But will it work in five year's time? Or when you've had a bad day? Or when you're feeling stressed?

Instead of saying, "I will just have to be restrained", think through the situation and plan exactly what you will be faced with and how you will deal with it, without feeling deprived.

How to Handle a Buffet

Let's talk through an example.

Imagine you're at a buffet dinner and there is a vast array of foods before you.

Your Plan A is to "Just be restrained" a.k.a. "I'll just be careful".

Plan B is to take a smart approach. Instead of trying to be restrained, you look over the buffet. In most cases, not every food there will be worth it. Some of it will be mediocre and other dishes will be downright bad. You don't want to waste your eating on mediocre or bad foods.

So look over the table and serve yourself only from the 2-3 dishes that you think really look worth it. Put everything you want on a plate, once. Don't go back for seconds.

Sit down and fully enjoy what you're eating. Savour every bite.

Sit as far away from the tables with the food as possible, so you don't feel tempted to reach over and get more.

Can you see that this strategy means that you will probably enjoy the meal more (because you're only focusing on things you like, rather than haphazardly sampling lots of dishes where the average rating will be lower)? But you'll also eat less, which is great, and it's a repeatable strategy, rather than the "just be restrained" strategy that could easily go wrong.

In this case, Plan A is foolish optimism, hoping that you'll somehow muddle through. Plan B is considered and sensible and much more likely to work.

Chapter Summary

1. Hoping for the best is not a strategy for coping with challenging situations.

2. Instead of foolish optimism, think the situation through and make plans.

19

SOMETIMES DOING
THE RIGHT THING
MEANS EATING CHOCOLATE

WHEN MOST PEOPLE HAVE A piece of chocolate, they can't stop themselves having one more and then another and pretty soon the whole bar is gone.

But for one of my clients (let's call her Isabel), this isn't a problem. She's able to have one piece and leave it at that. She's not the same with other foods – just chocolate. For some reason, she is satisfied with one piece. So for Isabel, chocolate is a perfectly acceptable snack.

Isabel is lucky enough that she can feel satisfied with one piece of chocolate. It's her strength and you should always play to your strengths.

How You Get Forced Into Denying Your Strengths

Sadly, for many years, Isabel had not realised it was a strength – in fact, quite the opposite. She felt that eating chocolate was a weakness that she should not be indulging in.

After all, every diet she had been on had talked about how bad chocolate was and to stop eating it. So when she did indulge, Isabel would feel extremely guilty.

This is one of the many reasons why diets don't work.

They are not personalised. They don't respect individual differences.

When you go on a diet, you're pretty much agreeing to follow the instructions no matter what. If you can stick to it, you're good. If you can't stick to it, you're a failure. But in those instructions may be directions that contradict or undermine your particular eating style.

This is exactly why a particular diet may suit your friend but may not suit you. You have to be aware of your unique strengths and weaknesses.

For Isabel, the ability to eat one piece of chocolate and be satisfied was a strength to be celebrated, not a weakness to be avoided.

Finding Your Own Strength

Here are some examples of other clients' strengths:

1. Being able to eat a handful of nuts and no more than that.

2. Having just one piece of bread and feeling content with that.

3. Being satisfied with one glass of wine and not needing any more.

Again, with each of these examples, other people would not be able to do these things easily, which is what makes them so useful.

You have strengths, too. You may not recognise them yet but they are there.

Look at the foods you like, especially snacks.

Sure, there will be some foods that once you start eating, you can't stop. But there may be others that are satisfying in very small amounts. If you find one of these, grab on to it and hold it close! It will be a huge advantage in losing weight.

Coming back to Isabel, once she had discovered her strength, everything was easy after that, right? Not at all.

Because the brainwashing from diets was very deeply ingrained, Isabel would be going along quite nicely and then suddenly start feeling guilty about eating chocolate and so try and cut back.

When she stopped eating chocolate, she would try and satisfy the craving with other foods. The problem was that she needed to eat a lot more of the other food to get the same effect of one piece of chocolate.

I had to keep reminding Isabel that eating chocolate was OK!

The other thing you need to be alert for is mistakenly thinking that something is a strength and then finding out that, actually, you keep eating more of it each day. In this case, you haven't found a strength, you've found a danger food. (More on that in the next chapter.)

But whether you find a strength or not, the underlying message you should take on board is that not all advice applies to everyone. Question it. Test it. See if it's true for you before accepting it.

And if you can, go for what feels natural.

Instead of feeling guilty for not following standard diet advice, do what comes naturally and it will be much easier to stick with it for the long-term.

Chapter Summary

1. Look for your personal eating strengths. There are foods that you can eat that don't get out of hand.

2. Instead of denying these strengths, celebrate them. They are your friends on your weight loss journey.

20

BEWARE THE DANGER FOOD

IN THE LAST CHAPTER I briefly mentioned the "danger food". If you've read my book *Slim and Healthy without Dieting*, you'll know what I mean by the term danger food; it is a food that is specific to you and it causes far more damage to your waistline than any other food.

It's hard to say no to a danger food. It's also hard to stop at just one serve.

And if you have a danger food on one day, you get the craving for it again the next day at the same time.

Examples of danger foods include chocolates, crisps and cakes.

But actually a danger food can be anything that fulfils those things I've mentioned.

The Surprising Danger Food

I had one client, let's call her Grace, whose danger food was satsumas (a type of citrus fruit). Grace could eat ten in a day and found it difficult to stop.

It had all begun in her dark dieting past, when she had been on diets that had stated she could eat as much fruit as she wanted. Grace was actually encouraged to eat them.

And what started as a crutch to get through a depriving diet became a danger food.

When Grace was eating satsumas, she lost control.

Of course, it seems ridiculous to suggest that something considered so healthy as fruit could be problem but they certainly were. And as I mentioned in an earlier chapter, fruit is not harmless. It contains sugar and hence calories.

But most conventional diets would not have a problem with Grace's fruit habit. Diets simplify rules down to be generic and fruit seems to pass under the radar, even if it's ten satsumas a day.

But my point is: regardless of what it is, when it goes from a deliberate decision to mindless eating, it becomes unnecessary. And the way that you lose weight with this approach comes down to eliminating unnecessary eating.

Interestingly, when Grace switched from satsumas to oranges (one citrus fruit to another), she was much more in control. It just goes to show how quirky food preferences can be.

How to Tame Your Danger Food

So, once you've identified your danger food, what should you do?

Well, if possible, you should eliminate it from your diet.

There are a few ways of doing this:

1. Go cold turkey. Just cut it out. Remember it's just one type of food and you can enjoy lots of other foods in its place.

2. Cut it down gradually. I find that a great way of doing this is to estimate how many you have in a week and then cut back by a small amount. E.g. if you have five packets of crisps per week, try and cut back to four, then the next week, three and so on.

3. It's ideal if you can replace the danger food with something else that you have more control over, so that if the situation arises, you've got something to eat, instead of having to turn to the usual. Remember your personal "strength" from the last chapter.

4. You don't have to eliminate the danger food completely. You could just make it a "special occasion" food or an "outside the home" food. That way you're not denying yourself but allowing it to become a special, but deliberate, choice.

Chapter Summary

1. You need to be aware of your danger food. These foods can be real problems if they are too accessible.

2. Best to indulge in other foods and either cut out the danger food or reserve it for special occasions.

21

THE WRONG KIND
OF OPTIMISM: PART 2

As we've just discussed previously, foolish optimism is when you avoid the hard job of thinking and try and fudge a casual response to challenging situations.

I have found that this often relates to snacks, specifically nuts.

I've heard clients say, "I will use nuts as a snack and just have ten of them". But nuts are as bad as crisps, in that it's hard to open a packet and just have ten. In many ways, it's worse with nuts; they are considered healthy, so they seem OK and you may feel justified in using them as a snack.

For most people, it really is a mistake to think that you can have a packet of nuts and each time you need a snack, be so in control as to take ten of them and then close the packet until next time (unless you have the gift of being satisfied with just a few nuts – see Chapter 19).

This might work one or two times but it is a slippery path. Nuts are just too "moreish" (you keep wanting more). Realistically, with nuts, you're faced with two alternatives:

1. Don't use them as a snack.

2. Use them as a snack but each time you buy a packet, be disciplined enough to portion them off into smaller containers.

With option two, be aware of another aspect of "foolish optimism": thinking that you will always be so organised and motivated enough to portion off smaller amounts.

There are some clients who are very disciplined about this and can manage it, but most clients will struggle with this in the longer-term. Either they never get around to buying the smaller containers, or they forget to do it.

But overall, whether it's nuts or some other food that you struggle to limit, don't just hope for the best. Have a plan and make sure the plan takes into account human nature and the tendency for eating to get out of hand when you have tasty, moreish snacks.

Chapter Summary

1. Some snacks (like nuts) are moreish. So you need to be careful with them.

2. If you do stick with them, you may need to develop a habit of portioning them off into smaller servings when you buy them.

22

THE GOLDEN QUESTION
DOESN'T WORK!

Remember the Golden Question?

"I can have it if I want to, but do I really need it right now?"

Every so often I will hear someone say something like: "Every time I ask myself the Golden Question, my response is 'Yes, I want it' and then I end up eating it. The question doesn't work!"

In other words, even though they're asking the Golden Question, they're ending up eating everything anyway.

First of all, the whole point of a "yes/no" question is that sometimes the answer can be "yes".

So there's nothing wrong with answering yes to the Golden Question. In fact, if you're not answering yes to it every now and then, then you're probably using the question badly and denying yourself foods that you might usually enjoy.

But equally, if you're *always* answering "yes", you're also using the question wrongly.

If you're always answering yes, it means you're following the first part of the question ("I can have it if I want to") but not following the second part of the question ("Do I really need it right now?").

How to Decide If You Really Do Need it Right Now

When most people see food, they ask themselves, "Do I want it?" and the answer is usually: "Yes, of course I do!"

But the Golden Question makes you think about eating in a different way. Let's look at an example to demonstrate how it can work.

Let's say it's 5 p.m. and your children are having ice cream.

If you ask yourself, "Do I want ice cream?" you could easily say, "Yes, I want it. After all, it's ice cream and I like ice cream."

But when you evaluate whether "Do I really need it right now?" you start to think of other factors that might influence the decision. Here are things you might consider:

Am I hungry? Am I going to eat later? Do I even like this particular ice cream? How much do I need to feel satisfied? How will I feel after eating this? Will I feel better or worse? Will I regret this decision?

These sorts of questions change the whole decision-making process.

Now it's not just a case of whether you want it but does it make sense to eat it right now? Or is it better to eat it later? Or give it a miss altogether? And if you decide to eat it, how much do you need to eat to feel satisfied?

This second part of the Golden Question is crucial. It is the reason why being able to eat whatever you want won't end up with overeating.

The Golden Question makes you clarify which foods you really love and how much of them you need to eat to feel satisfied.

When you introduce this awareness to your eating and practice it consistently (which is the aim of this approach), you will be able to enjoy food and manage your weight for life.

Chapter Summary

1. With the Golden Question ("I can have it if I want to, but do I really need it right now?"), it's OK to answer "yes"!

2. But if you're answering "yes" all the time, it probably means you're focused too much on the "I can have it if I want to" and not enough on the "but do I really need it right now?"

23

FOOD DIARY REVIEW #1: GETTING HUNGRY IN THE EVENING?

WE'VE COVERED A FEW IMPORTANT principles so far but it's always useful to see these ideas in practice. So, throughout the rest of this book, I'll occasionally take the opportunity to go through some actual client food diaries to illustrate how this approach works in practice.

Food Diary Review #1: Fiona

One of my clients, Fiona, sent in her food diary. Here is a summary of her evening eating, which are in my words, not hers:

5 p.m.: "Kid's size" portion of dinner

9.30 p.m. Feeling empty but not necessarily hungry

Although she felt "empty", Fiona decided to go to sleep instead of eating. Usually this would be a time when she indulged in wine and crisps.

There are a few points to make here:

1. Is it hunger?

Fiona described what she was feeling at 9.30 p.m. as "empty", not hungry. This shows that she is trying to figure out whether she is hungry or not.

If you always have chocolate at around 10 p.m. every night, then on a night you don't have it, you will feel some kind of desire for it; that may not necessarily be hunger but just missing out on a regular habit.

2. When do you prefer to eat?

I know that common advice is to not eat in the evenings. However it's not when you eat but how much you eat, that affects calorie intake. The problem is that there are many more opportunities to snack at 9.30 p.m. compared to 9.30 a.m.

3. Is the gap too long?

In Fiona's case, she had a light meal at 5.30 p.m., which is quite early. It's no surprise if she is hungry by 9.30 p.m.

4. Play to your strengths.

We talked about playing to your strengths in Chapter 19.

I have lots of clients who don't mind going to sleep feeling a little bit "empty". Others can't tolerate that sensation at all.

If you don't mind feeling that your stomach is a little empty when going to sleep, then that's a strength you should use; it means you don't need to eat closer to the time when you go to bed.

5. Is Fiona being a bit "diet-y"?

As I mentioned, eating at 5.30 p.m. and then expecting to last till bedtime can be difficult.

It comes down to Fiona's intention. Was she doing it because it suited her? Or was she doing it because she was trying to be "good"?

If she is not eating and feels deprived, then she is doing things wrong.

Remember: with this weight loss philosophy, we are talking about lifetime change. Unpleasantness is not sustainable.

Chapter Summary

1. Look at the timings of your meals and snacks in the evening. Are you eating enough to keep you going?

2. Are you able to go to sleep feeling slightly "empty". If so, that's great! Don't force food on yourself before you go to bed.

3. Don't push yourself to miss meals or go for long periods without eating if it feels unpleasant.

24

THE HEALTH HALO: STOP BEING MANIPULATED

Is ORGANIC FOOD GOOD FOR weight loss? How about fresh food?

And is food that is low in fat helpful for losing weight?

When you're looking at foods at the supermarket, the food marketers want to persuade you that certain products are good for you. But the conventional view of "good" doesn't necessarily match with what is "good for losing weight".

Earlier, I talked about how foods that were thought of as healthy (like fruit) were still high in calories and if you ate a lot of them (like the client who couldn't stop eating citrus fruit), you could gain weight.

In addition, terms like organic and fresh have a "halo effect". People start to associate qualities with these words that have nothing to do with the actual meaning.

For example, organic refers to the way in which the food is grown. It says nothing about calories.

Fresh refers to how recently the food was made or obtained and also the fact that it's not processed, tinned or frozen. Again, there's no implication of calories.

Low-fat is another classic halo word. Low-fat does not necessarily mean low calorie. Many low-fat foods are high in sugar, so the calories are the same or could even be more.

Here are some other variations of health halos to watch out for:

"Baked not fried"

"Less than 10% fat"

"Less than 6g fat"

"Fat-free"

Each of these examples makes no mention of calories.

The Low Calorie Halo

But what about low-calorie foods? There's no confusion there. Low calorie means what it says. Surely in this case there's no halo effect?

But actually, low-calorie foods can also have a halo effect.

When people eat something that is low-calorie, it makes them feel like they can:

1. Eat more of it.

Low-calorie can sometimes feel like a license to eat more. But when there is a small difference in calories between the low-calorie and regular food and you eat double the amount, then that can be disastrous!

2. Eat other things as a reward for having the low-calorie food.

For example, you could save 200 calories by eating a breadless sandwich and then have a 300-calorie cookie afterwards as a reward. The choice of a low-calorie alternative gave you "permission" to have a reward that undid all the good of the low-calorie option.

Next time you're in a supermarket or buying food, look out for any labels and the halo effect. Not only do many of these terms not actually indicate whether the food is low in calories but even if they do, by purporting to have a health benefit, it lowers your guard and makes you either eat more of it or reward yourself for "doing the right thing".

Chapter Summary

1. When you see a food that suggests some kind of positive attribute like organic or low-calorie, check yourself. Are you being influenced into eating more of it because of the label?

25

FOOD DIARY REVIEW #2:
THIS IS A BAD FOOD DIARY,
BUT NOT FOR THE
REASONS YOU THINK

THIS FOOD DIARY IS FROM a client we'll call Ruth.

3 p.m. Cake with friend

5 p.m. Hot chocolate

7 p.m. Large pizza with husband

If you're thinking like a "dieter", your first reaction would be: "You shouldn't eat those things if you want to lose weight!" But of course, this far into the book, you're no longer a dieter and you probably agree that you should be able to eat whatever you want and not feel bad about it.

And in fact, seeing a food diary like this makes me happy, because it shows that the client is not depriving herself.

The food diary I've included here doesn't include what Ruth ate for breakfast and lunch, so it is a bit misleading. This wasn't all that Ruth ate during the day! But what is life without being able to share a cake with a friend or go out for pizza with your husband?

I want you to be able to go out and enjoy yourself and eat foods that you enjoy. I NEVER want you to give that up.

Why This is a "Bad" Food Diary

But there is something wrong with this food diary and you can't spot it because I haven't given you all the information from the food diary.

So let's fill in some extra details:

3 p.m. Cake with friend "Didn't really enjoy it"

5 p.m. Hot chocolate "Only drank half, as too sweet and didn't enjoy it at all"

7 p.m. Large pizza "Ate it because husband wanted it"

Now can you see what's wrong here?

Ruth has made three mistakes here. But it's not about the foods themselves. It's the fact that Ruth couldn't justify any of these food decisions with a good reason. None of these food choices are nutritious. We can accept that. But in this case, the problem is that Ruth didn't actually want any of them.

In the first case, it was a cake that she didn't like. In the second case, it was a drink she didn't like but she still drank half of it. And in the third instance, her husband has influenced her decision and she has eaten a whole lot of calories needlessly.

So here's what I recommended to Ruth and you can try this too.

For the next week, you can eat whatever you want but only eat it if you absolutely want it and it tastes great. Don't settle for bad cake or mediocre hot chocolate. Don't settle for anything that you don't feel like or don't enjoy. Be completely ruthless about this for a week. If you're out somewhere, don't go along with what others are ordering. Get what you want.

If you're going to have the calories, surely you don't want to waste them on things you don't like?

Chapter Summary

1. You can have whatever you want but make sure it's actually what you want.

2. Be discerning. Only eat food if it's really worth it.

26

A SIMPLE TIP THAT
STILL AMAZES ME

THIS IS A TIP THAT has made a big difference to many of my clients. And I am still amazed at how well it works (even when I try it myself) since it's *so* simple.

You can use this tip when you're deciding whether to eat something or not.

Let's think of a few examples:

1. Someone offers you dessert (after a particularly filling meal).

2. You're tempted to buy a chocolate bar (after you've just eaten).

3. You are about to open a packet of crisps (although you know you're about to have dinner in ½ hour).

Notice that I have specifically mentioned situations where you really don't need to eat those things. In all of these situations you've either just eaten and are full, or are about to eat. You can't really justify eating those things and yet you have probably had situations exactly like these where you gave in to temptation.

A strategy to use in these sorts of scenarios is to *wait 20 minutes.*

Yes, it's that simple.

You are allowed to eat it. I've told you, you can have whatever you want. But just wait 20 minutes. If you still feel like eating it in 20 minutes, then go for it.

But what you'll find is, in more cases than not, if you wait 20 minutes, you'll forget all about the food, or not feel like it.

As I said, it's incredible how well this works.

The 20 minutes puts some distance between you and the decision. It stops the impulsive eating, which isn't necessarily associated with hunger. And with the delay, the impulse amazingly vanishes.

Stop Making The Same Mistakes

A variation of this strategy is to ask, "How will I feel in 20 minutes time?"

Your present-moment-you is faced with a decision but this question makes you consider it from the future-you's point of view. How will you feel in 20 minutes?

If you've ever eaten something and regretted it later, part of the disappointment is in making the mistake. But a part of it is also about making the *same mistake over and over again.* To break the cycle, you need to begin to make a strong connection between the consequences and the action.

For instance, if you know that despite the allure of dessert, you always feel bad afterwards, then asking how you will feel in 20 minutes is a way of making that connection. This forces you to think of what happened in the past and remind yourself: "Actually that's never turned out well".

The first few times you do this, it may not work so well. But the more you do it, the more you will be increasing your awareness of the consequences of decisions.

You'll see beyond the fleeting tastes and to the longer-term effects.

And it costs nothing in enjoyment, because you'll feel happier after the meal than if you'd caved in and overeaten.

Chapter Summary

1. When faced with an optional snack, wait 20 minutes before eating it. This simple tip will save you many unnecessary calories.

2. A variation on this is to think about how you'll feel in 20 minutes. The more you can make a connection between the present moment and the consequence of a decision, the more you will make better decisions.

27

MAKE IT DIFFICULT TO EAT

IMAGINE IF, WHEN COOKING SOMETHING for dinner, that each time you needed a new ingredient you had to leave the house, go to the supermarket, buy it and then come back.

Of course, you wouldn't do that because it would be a ridiculous waste of time and energy.

In most areas of life, we try and reduce inconvenience (which translates into wasted effort) by keeping things at hand. This makes sense in general but when it comes to snacking, the pursuit of convenience is a bad idea.

For example, imagine you're watching TV and eating crisps. It's certainly more convenient to keep the bag with you, so you can access them easily. On the other hand, if you have to keep getting up and going to the kitchen to grab a handful, it becomes annoying.

In fact, after a few trips to get some more crisps, it's almost not worth it.

Taking it a step further, if the bag of crisps wasn't even in the house but still back at the supermarket, meaning you had to leave the house to go and get it, then this is *really* inconvenient.

As you can see, making food inconvenient is a great way to reduce snacking.

An attempt to legally create snack inconvenience happened in 2012, when New York Mayor Michael Bloomberg tried to introduce a regulation banning super-size portions of cola.

Some people said that if the servings were smaller, people would just order two of them instead. But that is a misunderstanding of how human nature works. Sure, there might be some cola die-hards who would order two but the vast majority of people wouldn't. They would go with the default serving size.

For most people, it's too inconvenient to buy two and carry them around or go back and get another one.

The other thing we should remember with convenience is that having something available actually influences your cravings in the first place. For example, if you bought chocolate at the supermarket that day, knowing it's in the house may make you crave that particular type of chocolate after dinner, whereas if it wasn't in the house, you wouldn't have even thought of it.

Making things inconvenient seems to go against everything we strive for in our society. But when it comes to snacks, it's definitely worth making things more difficult to get to. The practical application of this is that you should be looking to introduce "helpful inconvenience" to your life in as many ways as possible:

"Make it a chore to eat more"

How to Introduce Inconvenience to Your Life

Here are seven ways to use inconvenience to your advantage.

1. Don't stock snacks that you like, at home. Buy them only when you get the urge to eat them.

2. Don't eat from the packet. Take a small portion and sit down to eat it. If you need more, go back and get some more. You may go back a few times but it's unlikely you will go back more than that.

3. Buy food in small portions.

4. At a restaurant, order less and tell yourself if it's not enough you can order more later. Most of the time you won't need more. You'll have saved yourself wasted food and calories.

5. Instead of driving around looking for a parking space closest to the store entrance, park further away and walk.

6. Don't eat in the kitchen.

7. If you take public transport, get off one stop before yours and walk to your destination.

Chapter Summary

1. Although we spend most of our lives trying to make life more convenient, when it comes to snacks and eating, aim for helpful inconvenience. "Make it a chore to eat more".

28

STOP GOING WITH THE FLOW

A CLIENT OF MINE (LET'S CALL HER CAROLINE) went for a business trip to Florence, Italy. It was a corporate gathering that took place every year.

The company that Caroline worked for was not particularly imaginative. Every year, they held this event in Florence (even though they weren't based there). And every year, the dinners were at exactly the same venues with exactly the same menus. Sadly, the predictability extended to Caroline coming back from her trip each year 3-4 pounds heavier.

But this year was different because Caroline was much more aware of her eating.

On the second night of trip, there was the usual meal at the usual restaurant, which included a pasta course served prior to the main course (In Italy, pasta is usually served before the main course).

The interesting thing for Caroline is that she didn't really like pasta. For her, if there was a choice between a pasta dish and a dessert, she would always prefer the dessert. And in previous years, Caroline would eat the pasta dish, simply because it was there and because everyone else was eating it.

She would feel quite full by the time dessert was served but then still eat dessert as well. And because she was already full, she didn't really enjoy the dessert.

This year, realising that she valued dessert more than pasta, Caroline gave the pasta a miss. This was an excellent decision, since there is no point eating something to which you are indifferent. It easily falls under the category of unnecessary eating.

By being aware, she not only ate less but also enjoyed the meal more.

How Much Un-Thinking Eating Do You Do?

You will have your own examples of un-thinking eating. Perhaps these sound familiar:

- Your friend orders a wine with dinner, so you have one too, even though you don't feel like it.

- Everyone is eating ice cream, so you have some even though you're not a fan.

- The set meal comes with three courses, even though you can't really eat three courses without feeling over-full.

A huge part of this process is opening your eyes to what you eat automatically without thought. This is classic unnecessary eating and the more you can eliminate this, the easier you will find it to lose weight.

Chapter Summary

1. With any food decisions, ask if you're just eating it because you're going with the flow.

2. When you eat things only because *you* want it (not just because everyone else is), you will save yourself lots of unnecessary calories.

29

WHEN NOTHING SEEMS
TO BE WORKING:
MASTERING THE
SEASONS OF WEIGHT LOSS

WHEN YOU LOOK BACK AT your life, you'll see that it seems to go in seasons. There are times when everything goes your way and you can do no wrong. At other times, no matter what you do, everything goes against you.

These seasons *don't* correspond to the actual seasons but they just reflect different times of your life, when things feel easier or more difficult.

What you may not have noticed is that there are "seasons" in managing your weight.

Weight-Loss Summer

When you're in weight-loss summer:

- Your hunger levels are lower.

- You don't feel cravings as much.

- You're satisfied with smaller portions.

- It's easier to resist temptation.

- You feel confident and everything about managing your weight feels easier.

When you're in summer mode, it is so easy to make changes to your eating. Motivation is high. Results come easily. Weight melts off. You achieve things that you never thought possible. Losing weight is fun!

When you're in weight-loss summer, be grateful and ride the wave as much as you can. Because as surely as there is winter every year, we should be aware that there will always be winter in weight management too.

Weight-Loss-Winter

In "weight-loss winter":

- You'll feel hungrier.

- Foods that you haven't craved for months will suddenly become tempting.

- Portions that once satisfied you, don't do it anymore.

- It's harder to resist temptation.

- There will be lots of social occasions that seem to derail your progress.

In weight-loss winter, even when you think you're doing everything right, your weight just doesn't budge.

Of course, this can be extremely frustrating. If you've experienced how good things can be in weight-loss summer, it's a real comedown when things become difficult and don't pay off in the same way.

But instead of struggling, wait it out.

Understand that things are going to be a bit of challenge and don't put too much pressure on yourself. You don't need to push ahead right now. Just consolidate. Make sure you're doing the basics right:

- Ask the Golden Question

- Control your environment. Don't let extra snacks into the house

- Make sure bad habits aren't creeping back in.

And take into account that you might be a little hungrier than usual and allow yourself that little bit extra, if it's needed.

As with the real seasons, even when you're in the depths of winter, you can comfort yourself knowing that summer is around the corner. And when summer comes, all these challenges will melt away.

When you're swimming in summer, it becomes hard to recall that the same water was freezing cold just a few months ago. And similarly, once you're back in weight-loss-summer, the challenges you faced in weight-loss winter will be a distant memory.

Chapter Summary

1. Weight loss, like life, goes in seasons.

2. Enjoy and make the most of weight-loss summer.

3. In weight-loss winter, bide your time, make sure you're doing the right things, keep on track and wait for weight-loss summer to come again.

4. Weight-loss summer *always* comes around again.

30

NO MORE GUILTY PLEASURES

ONE OF THE BIZARRE REALITIES of food and dieting is that, when a serial dieter gets a chance to have a food that they really crave, they don't actually enjoy it.

Serial dieters will often describe scoffing down food so fast that they don't even recall what it tastes like. This is because the object of their affection is filled with both desire and guilt.

When you're not allowed to have a particular food, your desire for it increases. But then consuming it is accompanied by guilt at giving in to the temptation. So even when you get to eat that chocolate you crave, you don't get to enjoy it.

At the risk of over-simplifying, here's my advice to you: Don't do this.

First of all, as I've mentioned throughout this book, no food is forbidden. You are allowed to eat whatever you want.

Secondly, if it is a food that you like, then enjoy it. Actually enjoy it. And this starts with the setting. When you are having a food you like, make sure you can give it your full attention.

The other day, I saw a couple of women in a cafe engrossed in a conversation about a difficult colleague at work. But while doing this, one of the women was rapidly eating a piece of cake. How can you enjoy a piece of cake while you're completely distracted by talking with your friend about your outrage?

How to Enjoy Eating

When you're eating something you love:

1. Give yourself permission to eat it. It's OK.

2. Make eating your desired food a deliberate decision. You never want to eat it just because it was there.

3. Eat while sitting down.

4. Don't eat while rushing, driving, getting angry or otherwise distracted.

5. Eat slowly. Savour the taste. Enjoy the textures and the aromas. Relish every bite. Remember this is a food that you love. You owe it to yourself to enjoy it properly.

Make eating food you love (or any food for that matter) an occasion. Give it the respect and time to really enjoy it.

When you do this you won't feel guilty and you won't feel compelled to stuff yourself just to eat as much as you can before it's taken away again.

The paradoxical result of this? You will actually eat *less* of the foods you previously couldn't resist. And you'll enjoy them more.

This might seem unbelievable to you but this awakening is something I hear from clients every day. It's always some variation of: "I no longer have cravings for all those foods I couldn't resist before".

It's worth trying out, isn't it?

Remember food is to be enjoyed. So enjoy it!

Chapter Summary

1. I want you to eat food you love. But in doing so, make it a proper, enjoyable experience. Don't eat in a rush and don't eat while distracted or angry.

2. Savour foods you love.

31

WHAT TO DO
WHEN SOMEONE
PRESSURES YOU TO EAT

I ONCE MET A PERSONAL TRAINER who told me he was very strict with his clients about their diets and exercise. If a client mentioned that they'd had a few alcoholic drinks, some chocolate or – heaven forbid – a slice of pizza, he would really let them have it.

As you can imagine, I don't agree with this at all. Not only is sticking to his plan quite unreasonable (and unpleasant) but you can bet his clients ended up not being particularly honest with him about their eating or drinking.

The problem is that dieting is all about instantaneous perfection. You have to switch from your normal pattern of eating to sticking perfectly to a regime, overnight. And not conforming to the ideal is viewed as failure.

But I believe that every aspect of losing weight needs to be practical and realistic.

And for many people, aiming for perfection ends up with them not sticking to the plan, feeling like they've failed and then giving up.

If aiming for perfection means that you end up failing completely, I think that is a poor outcome. I'd rather settle for imperfect progress than perfect failure.

I want you to aim for "good-enough".

Let me give you an example of this good-enough approach involving obligation eating. Obligation eating is where someone else pressures you to eat something you don't want.

This can be a very common issue and for some people it's a disproportionate contributor to their overeating.

In an ideal world, what is the best solution to someone else pressuring you to eat?

Just say no. Don't do it. Don't worry about what they think.

Ideally, you shouldn't be influenced by someone else's pressure and you shouldn't care how they respond.

But for some people, this is a step too far. They are fighting years of conditioning and it's really tough for them to ignore other's wishes.

If I was to expect someone to immediately jump to the ideal response of just saying no, it might set them up for failure, because it so far from where they are now. So sometimes we have to stop expecting perfection and be OK with imperfect progress to begin with.

Let me give you two examples from clients.

Example #1

Sadie had gone out for lunch with her husband and another couple. After the meal, she felt comfortable and had really enjoyed the meal.

She was very pleased with how she had handled the situation.

But she was caught off guard when her friend Anne suggested they stop at an ice cream store nearby for dessert. "You have to try their double sundaes," insisted Anne. Sadie found it very difficult to resist pressure from others. And Anne putting her in this situation made her feel very agitated and upset.

Sadie knew from our previous sessions that she needed to get better at resisting pressure like this but it was too hard to do in the moment, especially when Anne repeatedly said, "I really wanted you to try these sundaes". Sadie felt it would be rude to refuse.

But inside, she was very angry that she was being put in this situation.

It's easy for us to look at the situation from the outside and tell Sadie to "Just say no". But in the moment,

Sadie felt it was too difficult to say no and therefore felt compelled to go along with it.

Anne ordered Sadie a massive double sundae. Sadie ate the sundae as fast as she could, all the while silently cursing her friend for the pressure she was placing on her. When she finished the double sundae, Sadie felt doubly sick: sick from eating so much ice cream so quickly and sick from the feeling that she had undermined her progress by eating something so blatantly unnecessary.

Example #2

My client Juliet was out for lunch with her friend, Marilyn.

Marilyn was overweight and would often criticise Juliet for wanting to lose weight.

Juliet felt very uncomfortable talking to Marilyn about weight loss and found her comments undermining.

Now, of course, the ideal solution was for Juliet to ignore Marilyn. Who cares what she thinks? Juliet should focus on looking after her own weight. But this was difficult for Juliet. She was working on getting more resilient to this but at the time it was too difficult to address head-on.

After lunch they went for a walk and Marilyn spotted a mobile ice cream van. She suggested getting an ice cream. Juliet didn't want ice cream but felt uncomfortable "making a scene" by saying no (of course it's arguable whether saying no to ice cream constitutes making a scene but it shows how your beliefs can warp your appraisal of a situation) so she decided to go along.

But rather than get upset and undermine herself like Sadie had (in our previous example), Juliet decided to be a little more calculating.

Marilyn ordered a cone. Juliet ordered her ice cream in a cup so that Marilyn couldn't see how much she was eating.

They sat down. Juliet took what she described as "the tiniest amount of ice cream" on the tip her spoon and slurped it down as if it was a full spoon. After 10-20 minutes, most of the ice cream had melted and in total, despite maybe 50 "spoonfuls", because she had put so little on the tip of her spoon, Juliet had eaten maybe the equivalent of only one spoonful of ice cream. She then offered to throw away Marilyn's napkin, stuffed it into her cup of melted ice cream and threw it away.

What To Do When You Can't Bring Yourself to Say "No Thank You" (Yet)

In a perfect world, when faced with the situation of pushy friends trying to force ice cream on them (that they didn't want), both women in these examples should have said, "No, thank you".

But depending on your past way of dealing with things, this can be hard to do. And that's OK. It's something you can work your way up to. Eventually you will feel comfortable saying no and realise it isn't rude and doesn't cause an international incident every time you do so.

But notice how Juliet dealt with it in a way that was inventive (and slightly comedic) and very effective at getting through the situation without overeating. Whereas Sadie handled it in a way that was self-destructive.

Yes, the aim is to eventually be assertive and say no. But along the way, if it's too difficult to just say no, then don't give up. Just be a little more inventive about it!

The point here relates to obligation eating but it has a wider message. Don't be blinded by the need for perfection.

Although many health and fitness "gurus" preach about living up to an ideal, sometimes it can feel too far away and too intimidating.

So it's better to go for imperfect progress than perfect failure.

Chapter Summary

1. Aim for progress not perfection.

2. It's better to do things in a non-ideal way, as long as it sets you on the right path.

3. Even if you initially find it hard to say no to obligation eating, you can find ways to work around it, without it ending in unnecessary overeating.

32

THE TALE OF THE ANNOYING HUSBAND AND THE UNWANTED ICE CREAM

IMAGINE THIS SCENARIO (this is based on something that happened to one of my clients):

You're sitting at home after dinner, watching TV. You feel comfortable and you're enjoying the show you're watching. You're not hungry. Everything is good.

Then your husband walks into the room with a bowl of chocolate ice cream. He sits down next to you. As he is noisily slurping the ice cream, you have a sensation rising up in you.

It's desire...for...ice cream.

Before this, you weren't even thinking about ice cream. What's happened? Isn't it fascinating that even though you weren't hungry, simply seeing your husband eat ice cream has made you desire it?

He offers you some. So you end up having ice cream, even though you didn't want any.

This is by definition unnecessary calories. Afterwards you feel disappointed, because you know you didn't need it.

So what should you do to avoid this happening again?

I asked the women on my newsletter mailing list for their thoughts on how to handle this situation and here is what they said:

1. "Divorce him" (Yikes!)

2. "This is why I'm glad I'm not married"

3. "Have fruit salad instead" (although fruit salad can be high in calories too)

4. "Make him throw it away"

But the most common answer was:

5. "Ask him to eat it somewhere else"

And in fact, that was what I suggested to my client and it seemed to work.

But…

This only worked because her husband was amenable to this; that is, he was OK with eating the ice cream in the kitchen beforehand. Of course, as with any scenario, not every strategy will work with everyone. So here are some other options (including some reader suggestions):

1. Not keeping ice cream in the house.

If this is possible, it's great.

If you live with others, it requires convincing them that ice cream should become a "special occasion" treat rather than an everyday snack.

2. Stocking flavours of ice cream that the rest of the family like but you don't.

If your husband likes mint chocolate chip and you don't, great!

3. Not sitting directly next to your husband when he's eating ice cream.

It's more tempting if he's right next to you with the food. This is especially relevant for snacks like crisps.

4. Leaving the room (not so practical if you're in the middle of a programme that you are watching but then you can always record it).

5. Having something to eat (less calorific) while he eats ice cream. It's much easier to not eat what he's having if you're having something else instead.

6. Have a tiny portion of the ice cream, enough to get a taste but no more.

7. Delay, don't deny. Tell yourself you can have some, but later (e.g. in twenty minutes or tomorrow) (see Chapter 26).

Most people (who are dieters and don't know about this non-diet approach) would see this situation and say,

"Just don't eat it", which requires a cast-iron will. But as you can see, there are a number of ways of dealing with it that don't require willpower.

This is true of every eating situation you will come across.

Chapter Summary

1. Life will throw all sorts of different eating situations at you. You need to be thoughtful about how you will deal with them. "Just don't do it" isn't a strategy.

33

USE ALL THE HELP
YOU CAN GET

IMAGINE THAT ON THE WAY to an important meeting, your car broke down. You don't have time, so you jump out and start walking as fast as you can; but you don't think you're going to make it.

It's a disaster.

But just as you think all hope is lost, a friend drives up in her car and offers you a ride to where you're going.

Would you take the ride?

Of course you would.

Often when you're losing weight, circumstances will make things difficult for you, for example, a run of social events or a crisis at work. But at other times, circumstances will help you out. Just like a friend showing up at the right time to give you a ride, there will be situations that will make things easier for you. We are always looking at the long-term but in the short-term, if you can get a little help to reassess a particular relationship with food or drink, then you should grab the opportunity.

Let's go through some examples.

1. The Impending Wedding

I have a few clients who are in pre-wedding mode at the moment. They have children getting married in the next month or so and of course want to look their best.

Suddenly it seems easier to make the changes they need to. It's easier to consider your need for chocolate cake, when you know you're going to have to fit into that dress you've bought. The wedding provides an excellent opportunity to see how much you really need cake.

2. Lent

In case you didn't know, some people who observe Lent give up something perceived as a luxury for 40 days prior to Easter Sunday. This is a perfect opportunity to break the chocolate habit!

3. Staying With Friends Who Don't Drink That Much

If you're going to be staying at a friend's house and they don't drink much alcohol, rather than curse the friend's abstemiousness, use it as an opportunity to cut back your own alcohol intake.

It's not just about cutting back but also about asking: "Do I need alcohol to enjoy time with my friends?" That's how you parlay a short-term restriction into longer-term change.

4. The Supermarket Has Run Out Of Your Favourite Chocolate Ice Cream

Many nightly food rituals are just bad habits that you wouldn't start from scratch but are hard to kick. If the supermarket has run out of your favourite flavour, what a great opportunity to see if you can kick the nightly chocolate ice cream habit.

Life will throw these opportunities at you, which may offer the best chance to make a change that you otherwise might not have been able to achieve during your normal routine.

I should emphasise this isn't about demonising a particular food or actively ridding your life of it. But when you're in the grips of a habit, it's hard to see clearly. By piggybacking on another event, you get a chance to make some space where you can reassess your particular relationship with the food and set new guidelines for how you handle it.

Chapter Summary

1. Sometimes adjusting your relationship with certain foods or drinks can be difficult. When events like a wedding, Lent or even your supermarket running out of food, come along, grab them as opportunities to supercharge your progress.

34

DON'T BE GOOD

By now you should be comfortable with the fact that this approach is completely different to dieting. It involves a different mindset towards weight loss.

However, you'll find that diet-thinking is really hard to eliminate from your mind. I find that even clients who have totally embraced my approach to weight loss still find that old thought patterns persist.

Here are three examples of doing the wrong thing:

1. To make up for a heavy dinner the night before, you have a very light lunch. One that is so light, you still feel hungry afterwards.

Then a few hours later, you're starving. Someone has brought a chocolate cake to work for her birthday. You have three big pieces, because you're so hungry.

2. You get home and decide that, rather than having a full meal, you'll be good and just have some crackers. You end up eating ten crackers with cheese (which comes to more calories than a meal) and then because you don't feel like you've had something substantial enough, you spend the rest of the night picking at different foods in the kitchen.

3. The next night you go out for dinner with friends. While everyone is sharing plates of food, you virtuously decide to stick to a green salad. You get home later, starving and have a huge tub of ice cream.

In each of these examples, you've ended up eating more than you intended. And under these circumstances, you've lost control.

But what is the common link between all of these three decisions?

It's the thought: "I am being good".

When you think you're being good, you're probably going to make an unpleasant or drastic cut to your eating. If you ever have the thought "I am being good", then you've taken the wrong path. You've strayed into diet-y thinking. "Good" implies cutting back and feeling deprived. It implies denial.

The denial, as shown in those examples frequently leads to later indulgence. But instead of controlled, deliberate, enjoyable indulgence, it turns into desperate, uncontrolled gorging or binging.

Diet-based thinking is characterised by deprivation and unsustainability. Often, when you are trying to be "good", it means you think you need to feel deprived in order to lose weight. Of course this is not really the case.

Being good can also come up after a "bad day". When you get up the next morning, you might think: "Because I overate over the weekend, I need to be good today". But being good just compounds the problem, because the deprivation makes you end up eating more.

So after a bad weekend, what is the best response on a Monday morning?

Not denial. Not being good. Not thinking: "Oh well, what's the point?"

Instead, it's just getting back to the regular routine. Eating what you want but only as much as you want. Asking the Golden Question: "I can have it if I want to, but do I really need it right now?"

Remember: if you catch yourself thinking "I'm being good", you're actually being bad!

Chapter Summary

1. The thought of "being good" with your food and drink decisions shows you're heading down the diet path.

2. As soon as you catch yourself thinking "I'm being good", stop yourself and make sure you have a proper meal.

35

HOW TO HANDLE FLIGHTS

A CLIENT OF MINE WAS GOING on a long-haul flight from Europe to Australia. It was a 24-hour trip, with a stopover in Dubai. As you can imagine a long-haul flight can cause a few problems with your eating and drinking, including:

- Being tired.

- Using food as a reward for discomfort/tiredness/ boredom etc.

- The plentiful opportunities for overeating (especially when flying business class, which this client was).

- Getting into holiday mode and over-indulging because that's what you usually do on holidays.

Before I talk a bit more about this, consider how the average person who is on a diet approaches a plane flight like this one. This is the series of thoughts that may go through their mind:

"I'm on a diet."

"I always overeat when travelling."

"I don't know what to do."

"I'm going to gain weight."

"Oh well, there's nothing I can do."

"Ugh, I'm four pounds heavier!"

Most diets don't tell you how to deal with situations like this. And while you might not fly 24 hours to Australia every day, there are lots of other common situations that can undermine your weight loss efforts, like eating at a restaurant, going to the cinema, going on a weekend away, entertaining friends... The list goes on.

So with this client, we sat down and planned out every part of the trip. We made a plan to deal with all the potential obstacles and temptations. For example, one of the pitfalls of international travel, especially across time zones, is that you may end up eating four meals in a day. So one of the simplest things to do is to plan when your meals are going to be.

Will you eat at the airport, or on the plane? Will you eat as soon as you arrive at your destination? Or will you wait till mealtime?

I also often suggest taking along suitable snacks, so you're not at the mercy of only whatever is available.

A commonly known tip is to start living like you're already in the destination's time zone. So even if you get on the plane at night, if it's 2 p.m. in Australia, then start eating to that timetable. You should also include the layovers, stopovers and transits in your calculations of when you're going to eat.

It doesn't take too long to think this through and it will give you a lot more confidence about your ability to cope with the trip.

Now, of course, you can't anticipate every situation that might come up on a trip ("no plan survives contact with the enemy") but that's OK. You'll still be better prepared than if you'd just turned up and hoped for the best. As it turns out, for my client the plan worked very well. In a situation where others might have gained a few pounds, my client enjoyed the trip and gained no weight.

Chapter Summary

1. The plane trip is an example but you need to get better at dealing with all the eating challenges that come up in your life. Don't just hope for the best. Make a plan.

2. Make a list of situations that often end up with you over-eating and gaining weight. Examples include: Christmas, overseas trips, eating dinner at a friend's house.

3. Sit down and think through all the potential challenges. Make a plan to deal with the situation.

4. You'll find that simply thinking through the situation ahead of time will make it easier to handle.

36

FOOD DIARY REVIEW #3: MORE ON RESTAURANT EATING

IT'S TIME FOR ANOTHER FOOD diary review. This time let's look at Miranda's (another client's) food diary when she had dinner at a restaurant.

Breadbasket with butter – moved basket away from me so I couldn't reach it easily.

Starter: Deep-fried goat's cheese with a salad. Gave half to my husband.

Main: Baked salmon with French fries. Ate half.

Desert:. Chocolate cake with ice cream. Ate all of this. Probably didn't need to.

Let's go through some of the main points:

1. Although we tend to think of dinner at a restaurant as consisting of three courses (starter, main, dessert),

it's worth challenging this. Many of my clients find that two courses can be more than enough. Experiment with this and see how you feel.

2. Moving the bread and butter away was a good tactic.

Remember: "Hard to reach is hard to eat".

If something is out of arm's reach, you're much less likely to eat it than when it is right in front of you. This is such a basic strategy but most people either forget to do it, or think it's too obvious to make a difference. Trust me, it makes a difference!

3. Miranda was able to reduce what she was eating by sharing with her husband.

Sharing is always a good idea and you should do it as much as possible.

Just one thing to be aware of: Many clients tell me that when they share with their husband, they divide things up equally even if the husband is bigger and heavier than they are. That makes no sense! If the person you're sharing with is bigger than you, then they should get more. Dividing things equally is a relic from childhood, when, if another child was given more than you, you screamed, "It's not fair!"

Some clients have reservations about leaving more food or drink for their husbands ("He really needs to lose weight too!") on account of health concerns for an already out-of-shape partner. This is understandable but eating more just to prevent your partner eating it, is ridiculous!

4. If you can leave food on your plate, then that's ideal. Some people are able to do this quite easily. If you feel it's difficult to leave food, you are better off sharing. Miranda could have shared dessert with her husband and then her meal would have been perfect.

While there are lots of lessons in Miranda's food diary, the best lesson was that she was actively looking for ways to reduce her food intake (without affecting her enjoyment of the evening), as well as evaluating how effective her choices were.

Chapter Summary

1. When eating out, try having two courses instead of three and see if it works for you.

2. "Hard to reach is hard to eat" – keep food out of arm's reach and you'll eat less of it.

3. Share with others to eat less.

4. If your husband/partner is bigger than you, it makes no sense to divide up portions equally. They should definitely have larger servings than you.

37

DEATH BY CHOCOLATE SAUCE

Here's another story from one of my clients.

My client went out for dinner with her friend Jennifer and both of their husbands. My client told me that Jennifer was in her forties and had always been slim. At dinner, Jennifer ordered a starter and a main course. She also had a couple of glasses of wine.

She then ordered some profiteroles (a dessert like cream puffs) and asked the waiter for some chocolate sauce. The waiter obliged and began pouring the chocolate sauce on the profiteroles. My client was expecting Jennifer to say, "That's enough" after a small amount of the chocolate sauce was poured but she didn't.

In fact, eventually the bowl was so full with chocolate sauce that the profiteroles were completely submerged. Imagine a bowl filled to the brim with chocolate sauce (and some profiteroles bobbing around in there somewhere).

Remember, Jennifer is in her forties and slim. How does she maintain her weight, when she eats like this?

If my client had been anyone else, she would have looked on with envy, that Jennifer was so lucky to be able to eat this much and maintain her figure. But my client isn't like everyone else. She herself had lost over 30 pounds and other people now look at *her* with feelings of envy.

So my client, while slightly taken aback by the drowned profiteroles, could see exactly what was going on.

Do you know what was going on?

I asked women on my newsletter mailing list to tell me what they thought Jennifer's secret was. The responses included:

"Jennifer wears very tight fitting clothing to hide her expanding figure."

"Jennifer purges after eating."

"Jennifer is trying to tempt her friend into breaking the diet." (With friends like these who needs enemies?)

But the two explanations I was thinking of were:

1. Balanced Indulgence

My client was actually staying with Jennifer for the weekend and noticed that she ate very little before dinner that day.

If you have come across the term *balanced indulgence* in my other books, you will know that it is how women like

Jennifer give the impression to other women that they eat what they want and still don't gain weight.

In short, they eat more at certain times and balance it off at other times. For example, if you anticipate eating a heavier dinner, then you could have a lighter lunch (but not too light) that day. This is balanced indulgence and it's probably what Jennifer did that day.

2. Sharing

Jennifer had an arrangement with her husband for dessert. They would order two separate dishes and then share them.

But in practice, this meant that Jennifer enjoyed watching the profiteroles being submerged in chocolate but actually ate very little of the dish. She passed most of it onto her husband ("There's always a victim").

Her husband would finish off the rest.

So in many ways, the drowned profiteroles were just a bit of "indulgence theatre". They had nothing to do with how much Jennifer ate. All told, at the end of dessert, she had had a few mouthfuls, no more.

Of course, if you ever asked Jennifer how she remained slim while eating profiteroles drenched in chocolate, she would tell you something about her fast metabolism and good genes.

Don't believe it! After a certain age, people are slim because they practice certain habits. Jennifer looks like she is over-indulging but she's not.

Chapter Summary

1. When a woman over 40 appears to eat a lot but is still slim, it's not because of fast metabolism or good genes.

2. She is either practising "balanced indulgence" or despite appearances, she is not eating as much as it appears.

38

YOU'RE PROBABLY DOING BETTER THAN YOU THINK

WHEN I SEE CLIENTS AT my clinic, I get them to email me partway through the week with an update. A week can be a long time in weight loss, so it's good to touch base in between sessions to check what's happening.

With some clients, I notice that their mid-week emails often describe the previous few days as "terrible" and "really bad". When I see them later that week and look at their food diary and their weight measurements, I often notice that despite their alarming reports, they've actually *lost weight.*

On closer examination of their food diary, there may be a couple of slips but there are also plenty of examples of positive changes that have been made. For most people, it's a common mistake to focus on all the things going wrong and ignore all the progress they've made.

This doesn't just apply to their food diaries; it's how they live their lives.

It's like the picky single person meeting people and focusing on all the attributes their prospective mate doesn't have, instead of all the good things they do have.

As you go through this process and new behaviours become habits, it's easy to stop noticing the changes you have made. They will become second nature and your mind will be more focused on what isn't working yet. When you have a particularly "bad" weekend of overeating, it dominates your mind but you may lack the perspective to see it wasn't as bad as you thought and that it's far outweighed by the changes you made at other times during the week.

Sometimes, especially if you aren't weighing yourself daily, you might create a story in your mind that you've gained a huge amount of weight after just one bad day. This is why daily weighing is so valuable, because it is an instant reality check.

Some clients become so preoccupied with negatives that they start to convince themselves that they are failing when in fact the opposite is happening. To counteract this tendency to focus on negatives, look through your food diary and focus on all the positive changes you have made.

Some clients, when they're writing down what they ate for the day, also write down a comparison of what they would have eaten before they started my weight loss programme. It is a great way to remind themselves of how far they've come.

You must manage your attitude throughout the process of losing weight. Keep grounded and focused on all the positives, since you will find that they do far outweigh the negatives.

Catch yourself doing things right.

Chapter Summary

1. As more and more behaviour changes become second nature, it can be easy to not realise how far you've come.

2. We also have a natural tendency to focus on what's not working, rather than what is.

3. When reviewing your food diary, look for how much your eating has changed compared to previously.

4. Daily weighing also acts as a reality check to keep you on track.

39

THE CHALLENGE
OF FREE COOKIES

I SEE CLIENTS FROM ALL OVER the world and a person in Mexico City will share many of the same food problems as someone in Manchester or Melbourne.

Of course there are also differences.

I was reminded of this when one of my clients from the US (let's call her Olivia) sent in her food diary.

Went to the bank. Free cookies.

Went to an open home. Free cookies.

Went to a cookie store. Free cookies.

There are cookies everywhere! Wherever she goes, someone is trying to offer her food. Of course if you live in the States, you're probably nodding your head knowingly but here in the UK, although there is a lot of food around, it's unusual to get cookies offered to you when you're viewing a home to buy.

So, if you're living in the US, then my thoughts are with you, for all the food challenges you have to contend with every day. In comparison, everyone else has it easy!

So what did I advise for Olivia regarding the cookies?

The first thing is: when you're offered free cookies, don't automatically take them!

Ask yourself:

1. Do I actually like cookies?

That seems pretty obvious but I'm sure you've had situations when you've been offered food and without thinking you've automatically eaten it, even if you don't usually like that food.

2. If you like cookies, are the cookies on offer amazing?

As it turns out, the cookies at the bank weren't that great (I know it's hard to believe!). If you really like cookies, then you need to be discerning. If the cookies aren't that great, then why would you eat them? You can "use" your calories elsewhere on something worth it.

3. If you love cookies and the ones you get offered by financial institutions or estate agents really do taste amazing, then it's also a good idea to come back to the Golden Question.

You can have the cookies if you want to but do you really need them right now? If you've just had a large lunch and some dessert, then do you really need the cookies? If you're about to eat in 1/2 hour, do you really need the cookies?

4. Use the quality quota:

For foods you love, a quality quota can be very helpful. For example, you could set your quality quota at "three cookies a week". This means you can have *up to* three cookies in a week but they have to be amazing and it has to be a deliberate decision to eat them. This means you're setting a slight constraint on yourself but you're also giving yourself the freedom to indulge while ensuring that when you do so, it's worth it.

This makes a big difference compared to just saying, "I can't have them" or "I'm not allowed to have them", which sets up a vibe of deprivation. When you decide to eat one of the cookies on your quota, you need to eat it slowly and relish every bite. If you can't do that while standing in line at the bank, then don't eat them there.

The Worldwide Problem

I hope you can see that even if you don't live in the States, you will be confronted with food that is being offered to you and you have to make a choice whether to indulge or not. Use these criteria to be more discerning about your decision and avoid needless, extra eating, just "because it was there".

Chapter Summary

1. When offered food, ask yourself: Do I actually like this food? Is the food being offered, worth it? And ask the Golden Question: Do you really need it right now?

2. With foods you love, use a quality quota. Set a number that you can have each week but make sure when you have them, that you really enjoy every mouthful.

40

COMPARING YOURSELF
TO THE WRONG PEOPLE

YOU MAY HAVE HEARD THE saying "comparison is the thief of joy". It's usually directed towards the idea of "keeping up with the Joneses" but is equally applicable to losing weight. You are much better off focusing on yourself than trying to compare yourself to others.

Here are some key comparison mistakes:

1. Comparing yourself to your husband.

A common complaint I hear from clients is that when they and their husband decide to lose weight, their husband loses weight much quicker than they do. One client complained that her husband just had to look at food from a different angle and he'd lose weight.

Yes, it's unfair but men lose weight easier than women.

Men have more muscle mass and faster metabolisms. This means, if you and your husband are trying to lose weight, there's no sense in comparing how much you both lose. And certainly no sense in feeling discouraged if he loses weight quicker than you.

2. Comparing your current progress to the past.

When you were in your twenties, you could probably lose ten pounds in a week if you put your mind to it. But that sort of weight loss is not realistic after 40. For every single one of us, each year that goes by makes weight loss that little bit slower. So the past is irrelevant.

But equally, don't let this discourage you, because speed of weight loss is not important anyway. A 20-year-old can lose weight quickly but what's the point if they gain it all back soon after?

You don't need speed. You need weight loss that lasts. And that's available to anyone of any age.

3. The women on magazine covers are not people but artistic representations of people-like beings.

When the most beautiful women in the world have to be photoshopped in order to make it onto a magazine cover, you know that we as a society have taken a wrong turn somewhere. If you have ever seen a video showing the amount of "touching up" that happens to magazine images (including reducing the waist size of already stick thin models), then you know what I'm talking about.

These images are not real. So don't let unrealistic images corrupt your view of what you want to achieve in your life.

4. Comparing to someone after seeing them eat for one meal.

You can't watch someone else eat for one meal and ever hope to know what her true eating pattern is. Some slim women will eat one big meal and then compensate for it for the rest of the week (See Chapter 37).

Don't get depressed if you see someone who looks to be defying the laws of nature. Everyone pays the piper eventually.

5. Comparing your eating to overweight people.

One of the downsides of group-based weight-loss programmes is that being around people who are more overweight than you can make you feel complacent.

Similarly, I have had clients go to dinner with their very overweight friends and say it's not fair that the friends can eat whatever they want. To which I say, "Well, you could do that too, if you wanted to be overweight".

Yes, someone who mindlessly eats a lot of food has a certain kind of freedom. It's the freedom to be miserable about their weight.

The Ideal Comparison

Choosing whom you compare with is important, since when you make comparisons with someone who isn't like you, you can get unnecessarily discouraged and disillusioned. The ideal is to compare with no one but yourself. Your only aim should be to be better today than you were yesterday.

Chapter Summary

1. Don't compare weight loss with men.

2. Don't compare your weight loss with younger people or the younger you.

3. Don't think of images on magazine covers as representative of real human beings.

4. Don't compare yourself to someone else based on seeing them eat for one meal.

5. Don't compare your eating to overweight people. You can eat the way they eat if you want to be overweight too.

41

TWO FRIENDS MAKING ALL THE WRONG DECISIONS AT A CAFE

HERE'S A STORY OF TWO friends meeting up for a coffee. In this seemingly innocent encounter are a number of mistakes. See if you can spot them.

It was just before midday and Liz was catching up with her best friend, Joyce, at a cafe. They sat down and ordered a couple of skim-milk lattes. But just as the waitress was about to walk away, Joyce said, "It's almost lunchtime, shall we get something?"

"I'm not that hungry", said Liz.

"Let's just get a muffin then", said Joyce.

Liz didn't really like muffins but there didn't look to be anything else on the menu that she did like. So they both ordered blueberry muffins.

When the muffins arrived, Joyce had already launched into a tirade about an acquaintance of theirs. Caught up in the heat of the discussion, Liz didn't realise she'd polished off the entire muffin.

Commentary

Here's a list of mistakes:

1. Eating to time.

Do you sometimes eat lunch just because it's 12 o'clock? It's not a good reason to eat, just because the clock suggests it is "lunchtime".

2. Not listening to hunger.

How will you know how much to eat if you're not hungry? Liz wasn't hungry but still got dragged along with Joyce's choices.

3. Not thinking about the rest of the day.

Eating at just before midday would then throw off the rest of the day. Would eating the muffin mean they would skip lunch? It seemed unlikely. So it was just an extra (needless) hit of calories in the day.

4. Ordering something just because it was the least bad option on the menu.

Sometimes you can get in situations where you can't see anything on the menu and try and order the "least worst" alternative. It's doubtful whether muffins were the lowest calorie alternative anyway but it's doubly bad because Liz didn't even like muffins. Don't waste calories on things you don't like eating.

5. Not sharing one muffin.

Liz and Joyce could both have saved a lot of calories by sharing the muffin. It really wasn't necessary to have one each.

6. Eating while discussing something emotional.

As I mentioned in a previous chapter, when the topic of conversation is quite heated, it's best to avoid eating. You won't be able to appreciate the food and you'll end up just shovelling it down. It's obviously worse if it's a high-calorie indulgence.

7. Not savouring the muffin.

Of course, Liz doesn't like muffins, so she possibly wasn't that interested in savouring the taste. But eating it mindlessly is a very poor outcome.

What They Should Have Done

Let's envisage a better outcome:

They sit down and order coffees.

They enjoy the coffees.

They have lunch later when they feel like it.

Later on, they get a snack they actually want and eat it with total conscious awareness and enjoyment.

Ultimately, Liz and Joyce's tale was one of wasted calories. Assuming a blueberry muffin has at the very least 400 calories, they could have eaten much less, avoided 400 unnecessary calories and not missed out on any enjoyment.

And you can see that just a little bit of extra awareness about what's happening can totally change your experience of the situation and drastically reduce the amount of unnecessary calories.

Chapter Summary

1. Even in seemingly mundane situations like coffee with a friend, you can make small changes that mean you eat less, without feeling deprived

2. Don't eat to time. Just because it's "lunchtime" doesn't mean you need to have lunch, unless you're hungry.

42

HAS IT BEEN A GOOD WEEK
IF YOU DIDN'T LOSE WEIGHT?

CELESTE SAT DOWN IN FRONT of me at the clinic. She was very annoyed. This was her fourth session and since our last appointment a week ago, her weight was up.

Imagine that. You're in the middle of a weight loss programme. You get to the end of a particular week and your weight is actually higher than it was at the beginning of the week. In other words, while trying to lose weight, you actually *gained* weight

Is that a good week?

Most people would say, "No!" How can gaining weight when you're meant to be losing ever be good?

But actually with this approach gaining weight while trying to lose is very common and it can be a sign of progress.

Let's look at this more closely.

If you're on a diet, then it's definitely bad if you gain weight at the end of the week.

After all, with a diet, you're given a specific menu to follow and you're meant to start following it straight away. If you have gained weight at the end of the week, then you probably haven't been following the diet properly.

But with this approach, it's different. Remember, you're *learning* a new lifestyle and with any learning process there is an element of trial and error. For example, a child learning to ride a bike often falls over. You could argue that if your aim is to ride a bike, then falling over is a poor outcome. But it's obvious that falling over is a part of the process of learning how to ride a bike.

Gaining Weight After a Weekend Away

With Celeste, the reason she was heavier a week later was because she had gone away for the weekend and gained two pounds. But as we teased out the details of what happened, we could see some definite factors that contributed and we were able to work out a way to stop that happening again.

Yes, her weight went up that week but in the process she figured out better ways of managing her weight so that weekends away won't be so bad in the future. And the fact is, if you're someone who goes away for the weekend a lot, then you *have* to figure out a way to do that without gaining weight.

If you're going to be slim and healthy for life, you need to learn how to handle common challenging situations. If you don't, you'll either have to avoid those situations forever or each time you are exposed to them you'll gain weight.

In other words, numerical progress on the scales is not as important as learning. If you learnt to deal with a situation that you couldn't deal with before, then that is a good outcome, regardless of what the scales show.

In fact, I would argue, that long-term weight maintenance is impossible without having setbacks that you learn from.

It May Seem Obvious, But...

This all seems quite simple and understandable. You may even think I'm stating the obvious. But the moment when you step on the scales and notice that your weight is up, it never feels so obvious.

Instead there is often a rush of emotions including disappointment, sadness, anger, frustration and worry.

But as we know, weight fluctuates for plenty of reasons. And as we've seen with Celeste's example, in the process of learning how to deal with certain situations your weight may go up.

I like to use the example of driving from one town to the next and there's a section of the road that isn't sealed and has lots of potholes. That part of the journey is bumpy and unpleasant.

You might hate that part of the journey. You might wish it never existed. But if you're driving that road and you want to get to your destination, there is no way to avoid it. It is part of the journey. You certainly wouldn't turn back, because you know somewhere beyond the rough patch is your destination.

As difficult as it is, when you step on the scales in the morning and see that your weight has gone up, especially after a setback, it's important to learn the lesson from what happened, understand it's part of the process and not get discouraged. It's not pleasant but it's something you have to get through to get to your goal.

The right response, no matter what the weight shows, is to just keep going.

Chapter Summary

1. When you're learning a new lifestyle, trial and error means that there might be a few upticks in your weight. This is a painful but necessary part of the process.

2. It's worth it to have a small uptick in weight if you learn a better way to handle a challenging eating situation.

3. The right response to your weight not moving in the right direction is to just keep going.

43

DON'T FORGET
HOW YOU GOT HERE

Part 1: "It Should Be Quicker Second Time Around"

A client, let's call her Lucinda, who had lost about 20 pounds of weight and kept it off for three years, had been caught up in a crisis at work over a few weeks. Lucinda emailed me to say that during this time, her weight was up four pounds.

For the average person gaining four pounds is a disaster and often leads to giving up. For Lucinda, however, she had been doing this for three years and knew exactly what she had to do.

I felt reassured.

But then I got an email a week later from her saying that things weren't going well. She said that after a week, she had "only" lost one pound.

Lucinda was considering drastically cutting back what she was eating in order to lose weight quicker.

Interesting.

When Lucinda had originally lost weight, she had lost about one pound a week. This means that she was disappointed, even though she was actually losing weight at the same rate as previously.

Can you see what's happening here?

Although she had a great attitude and was able to get back on track after a setback, Lucinda was forgetting the original journey (which is understandable since it was three years ago). She was expecting to lose weight a lot quicker this time and therefore putting unreasonable pressure on herself.

If clients regain weight it is common for them to expect to lose it quicker the second time around. But of course, it's not rational. And when you create this kind of urgency, it makes you tempted to start cutting back drastically.

Lucinda did not cut back drastically to get to her goal in the first place, so why start now?

A better response, as Lucinda realised, was to remember that one pound a week was the rate she lost it at and to just aim for that. But even better, forget about the weight for the moment and focus on getting back to making the right decisions (keep asking the Golden Question). That's really what works.

Part 2: Fresh Fish

A client who had lost ten pounds with some gentle changes to her habits was on holiday. She had deviated from the plan and gained a couple of pounds.

When she sent me an update, her email said, "I've gained a couple of pounds, so I'm going to focus on eating more fresh fish".

What?

That's not how she lost weight in the first place! So why focus on these things now?

It's not a bad thing to eat fresh fish but it had not been the key to her successful weight loss so far.

Chapter Summary

1. Because this weight loss method is different to most, it can be easy to forget how you achieved success and instead revert back to diet-y thinking.

2. Try and remember the exact things that you did and how long it took to lose weight. Don't expect diet-y miracles when you didn't do it that way in the first place.

44

HOW TO MAINTAIN
YOUR WEIGHT LOSS

I VIEW WEIGHT LOSS IN TWO phases: weight loss and weight maintenance.

Diets focus almost exclusively on weight loss, so that even if you get to your goal, you are poorly equipped to maintain it. This is why people on diets end up losing weight and then gaining it all back. But if you've followed my approach you should have a different experience.

You should have only made changes to your eating that you're willing to do for the rest of your life so this makes weight maintenance easier. But even then, there are a few things you need to know if you want to maintain your weight loss forever and it starts with this:

The price of weight loss freedom is eternal vigilance.

What does eternal vigilance mean in a practical sense?

1. Weighing Yourself Daily

This is a habit that you should definitely retain, because it is your early-warning system for when things go wrong.

As I mentioned earlier, the reason I am so keen that you weigh yourself from the beginning is because I want you to be completely comfortable with daily weighing (and not freak out each time it fluctuates). This is so that by the time you come to maintaining your weight, you keep doing it for the long-term.

2. Checking In With Someone Regularly

Even clients who have lost weight and maintained it for years talk about the benefit of attending an appointment every six months or so. It serves as a focus, a reminder and a boost. It keeps them on their toes. Knowing they have to come and see me and update me on what's been going on, serves as a very useful prompt and ongoing motivator.

You also should try and find someone to check in with regularly. Maybe it's your family doctor or a friend. This will make a big difference to your ability to maintain your weight.

3. Being Extra-Vigilant About Your Environment

One of the common reasons for "blips" when you're maintaining your weight is not managing your environment properly. You need to prevent tempting foods from slipping under the radar into your home or office. The most common way for this to happen is via gifts from visiting friends. It feels wrong to throw out the gifts or to give them away but rest assured that keeping them in the house is a bad idea.

4. Beware Of Bad Habits Creeping In

It's so easy for bad habits to creep back in.

A client I saw recently had been having a small piece of fruit as a snack in the afternoon, when she was losing weight. But at her most recent appointment, the snack had suddenly turned into a cookie!

Another common one is the second serving at dinner creeping back in.

Or the piece of chocolate after dinner.

The beauty of having achieved your weight loss goal is that you know that you were able to manage without these little extra bits of food, so if they've suddenly appeared, it's clear that something isn't quite right.

But again, the difficulty is being aware enough to spot it. When you're the one going through it, it's hard to step back and see that these old behaviours have crept back in, hence the value of a second person looking at your progress.

5. Remembering Why You Did This In The First Place

It can be so easy (and understandable) that once you reach your goal weight, you forget the awful place you were in when you first decided to lose weight. Who wants to re-live unpleasant parts of their life?

But equally, if you forget how bad it was, it can sometimes lead to you devaluing what you've achieved. When we remember the past, it's easy to only remember the positives and get nostalgic. You might remember that feeling of being able to eat lots of food without thought. It becomes romanticised. You remember the good things and forget that:

a) It wasn't as satisfying as you think and

b) It came with a lot of negatives. In fact you were downright miserable.

It is better to be slim and healthy. If you've followed this approach correctly, you are not really missing out at all. You've just removed the unnecessary eating.

So there is nothing to be gained by going back to the old ways, no matter how much your mind might convince you that it'd be nice to eat like you did before.

Something that can help with remembering how far you've come is to look at old photos of yourself when you were overweight or to keep one item of clothing that is now too big.

It's How It Is

I hope the fact that you need to stay vigilant doesn't put you off.

I don't want to sugar-coat anything. This is the reality. It really comes down to trade-offs. If you want one thing, you need to trade something else. But when you consider the benefits of being your ideal healthy weight, staying vigilant is a small price to pay.

Chapter Summary

1. The price of weight loss freedom is eternal vigilance.

2. Weighing yourself every day is your early-warning system

3. Having someone check in on you can help keep you on track.

4. Watch your environment closely to avoid needless temptation creeping in, especially via gifts from friends or family.

5. It's useful to keep a reminder handy (like a photo or a piece of clothing) that reminds you what things were like when you were overweight. This is a prompt to stay vigilant and maintain your weight.

45

YOU CAN DO THIS!

W'E'RE REACHING THE END OF the book and my hope is that you can now see a path forward.

There *is* a way for you to take control of your weight and health and make lasting changes to your life. Your future is not one of powerlessness and feeling resigned to gaining more and more weight. You don't need to be a victim any more. Instead, you can take action and create a new, healthy relationship with food.

You can manage your weight, for life.

Words That Stick

Over the course of a programme of weight loss, I will say a lot of things to my clients.

It's fascinating to me, which things they forget and which become significant or poignant to them. It's often a throwaway comment that really resonates.

But there's one sentence that seems to have the biggest impact for the most people. I mentioned this in one of the earlier chapters and it's worth repeating again now.

"The only way you can fail with this approach is if you give up".

No matter what happens, with this weight loss approach, you can't fail unless you give up. What that means is, even if you have a "bad" day, a bad week, a bad month or even a bad *year*, it can't sink you. Unless you give up.

I've had clients who went AWOL for months, then came back, got back on track and achieved their goal.

So there is no reason for anxiety. Once you've made the choice to commit to this approach, you've made a powerful step towards freedom.

If you can't fail, then what will possibly stop you?

Expecting the Impossible

The issue will be unrealistic expectations. We have *all* been brainwashed by fad diet claims that we should be able to lose 10 pounds in 10 days.

We all think that a successful weight loss journey is one where the weight melts off.

We want the result as quick as possible.

We think that there should be no reversals, plateaus or setbacks. Any problems along the way mean either the weight loss method is faulty, or we are.

We expect to get on the scales and see that the weight has fallen some more, *every day*.

But it *never* happens that way.

Losing weight is, to borrow a common phrase, a marathon not a sprint. You won't be able to lose 10 pounds in 10 days. But if you're sick of diets and realise that they don't work, that won't bother you. Getting the result will be much more important.

This means that you will need to be determined and keep going, despite setbacks.

Because trust me, setbacks will happen. You're learning a whole new way of eating and drinking. You're reversing a lifetime of conditioning. Learning anything means making mistakes. And each time a setback appears, you will think something is wrong because we all expect our weight loss should unfold smoothly.

The reality is that weight loss should not be unpleasant or depriving but *there will be* plenty of reversals, plateaus and setbacks. As long as you don't quit and as long as you keep making small changes to your eating habits, you will keep making progress.

And if you keep making progress, then what can stop you?

No matter how discouraged you get (and there will be times when you will feel very discouraged; it happens to everyone), you have to remind yourself that you have the control. And you can persist.

The good news is that persistence is a habit. It's like a muscle that gets stronger and stronger each time you use it. Each time you overcome a setback and get back on track, it becomes easier to do next time. You can keep going, no matter what.

This is the key to success.

Remember: *"The only way you can fail with this approach is if you give up"*.

So... DON'T GIVE UP.

You can do this!

46

BRINGING IT ALL
TOGETHER

IN THE INTRODUCTION, I TOLD YOU that the value of this book was not just reading it through once but coming back to it regularly. I also think it's useful to summarise everything we've covered so far, so you've got a quick reference to come back to when you need it. So here's the summary.

1. Being fed up is good.

Although it's not great to feel fed up, often it's what needed so that you can throw out the old (diet) ways of thinking and embrace a totally new approach.

This is the first step to taking control.

2. Blaming yourself is bad.

Although you might feel that struggling to lose weight is your fault, I believe that much of your difficulty is because you tried to lose weight by dieting. And dieting doesn't work.

3. Change your focus to being slim for life.

When you focus only on losing weight, you will do short-term things like dieting. As soon as you stop the diet, you will gain back weight. Instead, think about how you can lose weight *and* keep it off.

4. Avoid deprivation.

If you feel deprived, you may be able to stick to the plan for a while but certainly not forever. The best long-term plan is one where you don't feel deprived.

5. Don't avoid social situations.

Instead of only trying to lose weight when your social schedule is empty, you need to learn how to handle all the different situations in your life and still maintain your weight. This means, for example, knowing how to manage eating when you go out for dinner or go on holiday.

6. The food diary is your friend.

A food diary is *the* essential tool for weight loss. It helps you know what's going on, guides your decision-making and can help you see what areas need improving.

7. Focus on changing habits.

Repeating a behaviour over and over again helps it to become a habit. But the habits that last are ones that fit into your lifestyle. This means making behaviour changes that are easy to live with. Don't do anything that is unpleasant.

8. It's good when things go wrong

When you're trying to lose weight and things go wrong, don't get down about it. It's an opportunity to learn a better way to handle the situation. You won't improve without this.

9. Use the Golden Question.

The Golden Question, "I can have it if I want to, but do I really need it right now?" is something you can ask yourself before every food or drink-related decision.

10. Eliminate unnecessary eating.

The way you can eat less without deprivation is to eliminate unnecessary eating. If eating something provides neither nutrition nor enjoyment, then it's unnecessary.

11. Remember that nothing is forbidden.

As soon as you say, "I'm not allowed to eat that", your cravings for it increase. On the other hand, if no food is forbidden, you'll be surprised at how much less you crave certain foods.

12. Aim to lose weight for the right reasons.

You don't need to lose weight to prove what kind of person you are. You're OK regardless.

13. Weigh yourself daily.

Weighing yourself daily is a very useful habit to develop. But the key is to not get too affected by the usual day-to-day fluctuations in weight.

14. Guard your environment.

The key to reducing temptation is not willpower but removing needlessly tempting foods from your surroundings. Make eating something indulgent a deliberate choice, not just because "it was there".

15. Buy what you don't like.

When you need to buy tempting foods for your family, buy flavours that they like but that you don't.

16. Out of sight, out of mind.

If you have tempting food at home, keep it out of sight. As soon as you see it, you will have a conversation with yourself over whether to eat it or not. Prevent that conversation from happening by not keeping it out in the open.

17. Reduce your portion sizes.

Ultimately, you need to cut back the portion sizes that you eat but the big mistake is to go too fast. Take it slowly. Start off even as low as cutting back 5%.

18. Don't make excuses or be a victim.

There will be lots of eating situations where it may be easy to just say, "There's nothing I can do". Don't think like this. There is always something you can do. Be proactive and never make excuses for overeating. Never act like you're a victim of circumstance.

19. Learn how to eat at a restaurant without overdoing it.

When going out for dinner, focus on the non-food aspects of the meal to shift the emphasis off trying to eat as much as possible.

20. Find your personal strengths.

There is a food out there, that you can eat a small amount of and feel satisfied, in a way that others can't. Find that food. It will be very helpful in your weight-loss journey.

21. Be aware of your danger food.

A danger food is one that you find difficult to eat in moderation. In these cases, it may be more useful to indulge in other foods instead or make it a special occasion food.

22. Ask the Golden Question properly.

If you find that the Golden Question isn't working, it's probably because you're focused on the first part of the question ("I can have it if I want to") but not the second part ("But do I really need it right now?").

23. Look at your meal schedule.

Are you eating too often or leaving too long between meals (so you are over-hungry by the time you get to your next meal – and then end up overeating)?

24. Remember that you're learning a new lifestyle.

When you learn to ride a bike, it's normal to fall off a few times. Learning a new eating lifestyle will also involve a few mishaps along the way. Don't let these discourage you. They are part of the process.

25. Beware the health halo.

If you feel you're eating something because of the food label (like "fat-free" or "low carb"), then make sure you're not influenced to over-eat. When you feel it has a health benefit, you're liable to eat more of it, or reward yourself for your "healthy" choice with a high-calorie snack afterwards.

26. Be discerning.

When you're indulging, only eat food that is amazing. Don't waste calories on mediocre food or food that you don't love.

27. Give it 20 minutes.

When deciding whether to have a snack or not, try waiting 20 minutes before having it. In most cases, you won't feel like it after the time has elapsed.

28. Give it 20 minutes: Part 2.

Think about how you'll feel in 20 minutes after you've eaten something. If you know that you'll probably regret it, then do something else instead. The more you can ask this question, the more you will make connections between present actions and future consequences.

29. Make it a chore to eat more.

Rather than making food conveniently available, try and put as many barriers as you can between you and food. Aim for "helpful inconvenience".

30. Don't go with the flow.

Often it's easy to get swept up with what everyone else is doing and eat things you don't even like. It's important to step back and stop yourself eating unnecessary calories in this way. Only eat food that you really want, not just because others are eating it.

31. Be aware of the seasons of weight loss.

Sometimes weight loss is easy (weight-loss summer). Other times it's really difficult (weight-loss winter). Your weight loss journey will go through seasons. Don't be too discouraged when times are tough, because easier times are always around the corner.

32. Enjoy food.

Most dieters eat food they love quickly and don't really enjoy it because they feel guilty. But you don't need to feel guilty at all. You're allowed to eat whatever you want. When you do eat foods that you really love, make sure to take the time to enjoy them.

33. Don't aim for perfection.

When you aim for perfection, you're probably going to be disappointed. I'd prefer you to make changes to your eating that are less than perfect but that you know you'll be able to stick with for the long-term.

34. Resist obligation eating.

In different situations, there will be people who try and force you to eat even when you don't want to. It's important to practice ways of resisting this.

35. Don't be good.

Any time you catch yourself having the thought "I'm being good", it means you're probably depriving yourself.

Don't do it. Aim to have proper meals and avoid being excessively hungry.

36. Think ahead.

Sometimes when a challenging eating situation approaches, it's useful to take a minute or two and make a plan for how to deal with it. Think of potential challenges and how you will sidestep them. This is much better than just showing up and hoping for the best.

37. Two courses, not three.

When out for dinner, most people are satisfied with only two courses.

38. Hard to reach is hard to eat.

It might seem ridiculously simple but keeping food out of arm's reach on the table will mean that you eat less of it.

39. Sharing is your friend.

The best way to sample a food without eating excessively is to share with others. Look for opportunities to share wherever you can.

40. Sharing doesn't have to be fair.

If your partner is bigger than you, you shouldn't be dividing up portions equally. They should be having more than you.

41. Balanced indulgence.

When someone looks like they eat a lot and are slim, it's because they're practicing balanced indulgence. They balance off a big meal with eating less at other times.

42. Don't automatically accept free food.

When you get offered free food, firstly ask yourself if you actually like the food (for example, if you don't like cookies, then don't eat a free cookie!). And secondly, is the food being offered good quality and worth eating?

43. Use the quality quota.

With foods you love, set a particular number you can have each week. Then you don't miss out but you have a limit to work to. Also, make sure when you do have them, that you really enjoy every mouthful.

44. Be careful whom you compare yourself with.

It's easy to get discouraged by comparing your weight loss to the wrong people. Remember: men and younger people will lose weight faster.

45. Weight-loss speed is irrelevant.

As long as you lose the weight and keep it off, that's all that matters.

46. Don't waste calories while emotional.

If you're angry about something, it's likely that when eating, your mind is going to be preoccupied with emotions and you won't fully enjoy the food. This is a waste of calories!

47. Patience is crucial.

Often when losing weight, progress will be slower than you thought. Most people get discouraged. But this is where patience is so important. Stay on track and the results will come.

48. Long-term weight success requires effort.

Compared to starting a new diet every few weeks, the effort required to maintain your weight will be minimal. But you still need to stay aware of your eating and your environment.

The price of weight loss freedom is eternal vigilance.

49. You can do this!

Weight loss should not be depriving or unpleasant but the reality is that there will be plenty of setbacks, reversals and plateaus. Expect things to go wrong. Accept it. And just keep going.

Remember, *"The only way you can fail with this approach is if you give up"*.

ABOUT THE AUTHOR

Dr Khandee Ahnaimugan is a medically qualified weight loss expert and bestselling author based in London, England.

Dr Ahnaimugan's clinic is based in London's Harley Street, where women over 40 from all over the world see him to learn how to lose weight without dieting or deprivation.

For more information visit:

www.DoctorKWeightLoss.com

FURTHER READING

IF THE WEIGHT LOSS APPROACH in this book makes sense to you, it's time to read Dr K's step-by-step guide to losing weight without dieting:

Slim and Healthy without Dieting: The Weight Loss Solution for Women over 40

For more practical examples of how to apply this approach to your life, read:

Losing Weight After 40: How to Change Your Life Without Dieting or Deprivation

21975962R00127

Printed in Great Britain
by Amazon